I0027087

CHOOSING TO
LIVE
WHEN TOLD TO
D.I.E

A MEMOIR

My Painful Journey Through
Deep Infiltrating Endometriosis

Crystal L. Brown

Copyright © 2023 by Crystal L. Brown

All rights reserved. No portion of this book may be reproduced or used in any manner without written permission of the copyright owner except as permitted by U.S. copyright law. For more information and permission requests, contact: 2275 Marietta Blvd NW, Suite 270326, Atlanta, GA 30318 or crystalbrown_1@outlook.com.

For privacy reasons, some names, locations, and dates may have been changed.

First Edition

Book design by Mary Ann Smith

ISBN 979-8-9891330-7-9 (hardcover)

ISBN 979-8-9891330-1-7 (paperback)

ISBN 979-8-9891330-0-0 (ebook)

ISBN 979-8-9891330-2-4 (audiobook)

www.crystalbrown.me

To women, the strongest creatures on the planet.

To Allen, who heated my blankets when I needed them most.

To both my miracles, Mommy loves you.

To Mom, thank you for everything.

In loving memory of my grandparents, Clarence and Nellie Ree Satcher.

I hope to make you proud.

CONTENTS

"Life is strange with its twists and turns
as every one of us sometimes learns."

-Edgar A. Guest

AUTHOR'S NOTE
Silent but Loud

It is our nature as human beings to criticize and review our lives when something terrible happens to us; questions form: *What did I do wrong? Am I a good person? Why me? Maybe too many drinks? Maybe that one cigarette? Maybe I was too harsh on my family or colleagues?*

"Why me?" lands the hardest. It lingers. It can haunt you if you let it. I toyed with this question for a long time before a still, small voice told me to write this book. Without my personal journey, I would not have been brave or bold enough to speak on the issue at all.

In middle school, I was in Upward Bound, a program for inner-city children who only had one way to go: up. Before we moved on to high school, our coordinator lined us up by height for the graduation ceremony. The agenda included a song and a poem. I don't remember the song, but I do remember the poem. An hour each day, my graduating class recited it until it stuck. Though I never admitted it to my peers back then, I was proud to recite it. Over two decades later, I still know it:

Don't Quit
by Edgar A. Guest

When things go wrong, as they sometimes will,
When the road you're trudging seems all uphill,

When funds are low and the debts are high,

And you want to smile, but you have to sigh,

When care is pressing you down a bit—rest if you must, but don't you quit.

Life is strange with its twists and turns.

As every one of us sometimes learns.

And many a fellow turns about, when he might have won had he stuck it out.

Don't give up though the pace seems slow—

you may succeed with another blow.

Often the struggler has given up,

when he might have captured the victor's cup;

and he learned too late when the night came down,

how close he was to the golden crown.

Success is failure turned inside out—the silver tint of the clouds of doubt,

and you never can tell how close you are,

it may be near when it seems afar;

so stick to the fight when you're hardest hit—

it's when things seem worst,

you must not quit.

I didn't know then—my innocent adolescent body un-assaulted; my soul unafraid and carefree; my spirit, content—that those words would present themselves repeatedly throughout my young life for, as I write this, I have undergone:

> a colonoscopy
> exploratory surgery
> one major surgery
> one hospitalization
> experimentation with a newly released drug
> the intake of an unknown number of pain pills
> an unknown number of antibiotics
> infinite tears

...all because of endometriosis. This disease came into my life—sudden, accelerated, wreaking havoc out of the gate—before I could get my bearings. It would present itself as the biggest fight of and for my life, and each day I had to choose not to quit. Any woman suffering from this excruciatingly painful illness would likely define it as hell. According to the World Health Organization (WHO), the medical definition of endometriosis is a disease in which tissue, similar to the lining of the uterus, grows outside of it. It can cause severe pain in the pelvis and make it harder to get pregnant. There are four stages of endometriosis—minimal; mild; moderate; and severe—depending on how extensive it is in the body. I was at stage 4: severe.

Endometriosis is silent but loud ... silent, because those whose bodies it inhabits often suffer in silence, but the pain that comes ... it is loud—excruciating—not just physically, but mentally, emotionally, socially, and financially. According to scholarly articles by medical professionals, the standard treatment includes two paths: (1) non-invasive: taking pain pills and birth control to manage symptoms; and (2) invasive: having laparoscopic surgery to diagnose and remove the lesions, or having a hysterectomy. Endometriosis impacts 10% of women globally (an estimation of about 189 million). In this book, I refer to endometriosis as endo, for short. My hope and prayer is that, through my story about the short- and long-term impacts this disease has had on my quality of life, awareness will be brought to the world about the girls and women suffering in silence in hopes that someone would become an advocate and ally for them—it could be you; the woman who suffers might even be someone you know.

I speak as one of the millions of women struggling with a disease with an unknown genesis. Thank you, for by reading this book, you are supporting our community.

— *Crystal*

1

FROM PARADISE
TO HELL

I spent the evening before my 32nd birthday at home, on my couch, sweating profusely. I lay still, wrapped in three heated blankets with two heat packs on my belly, avoiding any movement of my lower body. I waited for the alarm I had set to go off every three hours so I could take another round of 1000 mg of Tylenol and, three hours later, take 600 mg of Motrin— the best my doctor and surgeon could offer for relief. I had spoken with them at 3a.m that morning when I'd thought I was going to die. I felt the desire to avoid all birthday calls and text messages on the day I was born for fear I might break into tears. That cut the most. Why had I been born? Why should tomorrow feel special?

What I have presented is not my best image, so let me tell you more about my life before then. I was living in New York City, working for a fintech company during the tech start-up era, living a life I couldn't have dreamed of. I had worked in banking and consulting for the last ten years, traveling all over the country implementing software projects for financial institutions. I had had the #1 project in the company that year and the fastest project implementation the prior year. When the company needed someone to implement a new product, I was chosen to lead the team. I loved to get up in the morning, do my job, then work late and read up on my industry after hours. I had also been married for three years at that point. My husband, Allen, and I worked extremely hard. (We are cut from the same cloth and have similar upbringings, so we understand each other well. He is my partner and best friend.) We wanted to be successful and didn't let anything get in the way of that. We stayed up many late nights together either studying and/or working. At that point, there hadn't been many obstacles I couldn't overcome or strategize a way out of. I had grown up in the inner city of Birmingham, Alabama, where many are a population left behind. My hometown breeds resilient people. Through troubled times, I was taught by my mom and grandparents to grit my teeth and keep pushing until I came out the other side. I share this to give you an idea of how tough I had to be to get to where I was. I thought I had everything under control—until June 5th, 2018.

Allen had graduated from Columbia Business School's Executive MBA program a month prior, so I had been planning his graduation trip and our 2nd honeymoon (as I liked to call it) over the past 6 months. I had picked locations as far away from New York as possible: Singapore and Bali. Our trip was almost free because of the rate Allen and I had moved over the first two years of our marriage. We had traveled domestically and abroad for work, all while Allen had been in school nearly full-time. *We deserve this trip*, I thought, *so we are going to make the most of it!*

I dreamed about it every day—then finally, we were on a flight to Singapore after a layover in Paris. Life couldn't get any better, right?

But, on the flight, while everyone else was asleep, I wasn't. Oddly, my stomach was bloated, bubbly. I was relieved when we finally landed.

Allen and I had a great first day sightseeing and exploring the attractions; we spent one night in Singapore. The next day, we went to the airport to catch our flight to Bali. We arrived in paradise in the late evening and took the shuttle to our hotel, where we were offered a welcome wellness drink with local fruit. We signed a few forms and crashed for the night.

Around 5a.m. Indonesian time, I woke with an unusual urge to go to bathroom. Allen was still asleep.

It was late in the afternoon back home, so I called one of my friends while I sat, talking and laughing with her. I sat for nearly an hour. Although nothing was happening, my belly felt strange the entire time. *So odd*, I remember thinking. I figured my belly was adjusting to the Southeast Asian food and water.

Around 8a.m., Allen and I went to breakfast. The views were breathtaking, but breakfast was a blur. I didn't tell Allen I felt uneasy. I didn't want to ruin our trip. I ate very little, unsure of what would upset my stomach. When we returned to the hotel room, I couldn't hold out any longer—the growing pain was unimaginable. I told Allen I had lower abdominal pains, that something didn't feel right. Seconds later, I knew something was very, very wrong. I ran to the bathroom, wondering if water was trickling from my bottom. It was *diarrhea*. Frightened, I began to shake. I couldn't stop shaking. Over the next two days, I ran back and forth to the toilet about 25 times a day. My stomach had always seemed sensitive, but this was different—extremely different.

After day one in Bali, my cycle started. I assumed, due to the pain I felt, that somehow my body had kickstarted my period earlier than expected. But I was in such agonizing pain that, at 3a.m., Allen called the front desk hotel staff and asked that an on-call doctor to be sent to our room as soon as possible. The resort's manager, the doctor, and her assistant arrived in our suite within an hour to find me balled into a knot, trying not to move, drenched in sweat. The doctor was friendly but somewhat at a loss as to what the problem might be. She asked me to lay on the couch, then proceeded to check my abdomen—now the size of a basketball—with pushes and thumps. She prescribed some antibiotics and charcoal pills for the bloating and diarrhea. She was convinced, though, that it wasn't a food-borne illness.

Later, while Allen was asleep, I feverously searched the internet and found an Indonesian illness called Bali Belly. I thought I had discovered the root cause of my troubles. I hadn't.

For the next four days, I felt extremely weak. I had no appetite, no interest in social activities, and I looked six months pregnant. Leaving the resort for any reason felt like death by 1000 stabs to the pelvis. After the next two days, the symptoms subsided and I assumed the medicine was finally working. Allen and I enjoyed the remaining few days of our trip before boarding a plane to return to NYC. Little did I know, that was only the beginning.

One month later the diarrhea returned, but this time, with a fluid that appeared to be mucus. I went online and frantically searched for doctors who took appointments on a holiday. On July 4th, instead of being on Governor's Island or at Brooklyn Bridge Park basking in the sun sipping wine with friends, I had a brief visit with a local gastroenterologist in Brooklyn. I told him I had been in a foreign country, that my stomach was agitated and my bowels were producing mucus, not stool. He asked where Indonesia was, which made me feel uneasy, and his demeanor was nonchalant. He prescribed a stool test and a complete colonoscopy and sent me on my way.

As I waited outside for an Uber to take me home, I saw the doctor waving to a Range Rover waiting for him, jump in, and speed away. I stood still a few moments soaking in the fact that I still didn't know what was plaguing me and I had seemingly just wasted precious time with a provider who seemingly couldn't care less. I changed my mind about the Uber and walked to the nearest train station defeated, confused, with no answers and more questions.

The stool test was unpleasant, but I got it done and dropped it off, hoping the results would determine what medicine could eliminate ... whatever *this* was. Two weeks later, I received a call from the doctor's receptionist. In the typical hurried New Yorker voice, she said the stool test results had come back normal but to prepare for a complete colonoscopy. I told her I wanted to hold off on scheduling the appointment. Though the news was promising, my symptoms had subsided, and the coast was clear, deep down I felt uneasy.

Two months had passed; it was summertime. I was feeling incredible but my cycle was late, so I went to Target to pick up a pregnancy test. I peed on the stick and let it sit. (Was I ready to be a mom? How would I tell our family?) I ran a bath, relaxed, and read a book. After a time, sweaty and hot, I got out of the water and looked at the pregnancy test. I wasn't pregnant. I had known that was probably the case, but I had had to check because I was never late. I had been off the pill for a few months. *Maybe that was the cause of those unusual events over the last few months,* I thought.

One of my closest friends had called me a few months back and shared that she and her family would be in New York City for a wedding in August. Excited, I planned to visit them while they are in town. My friend arrived with her hubby and son, and I rented a car to drive over and pick her up. Before we left, her hubby wanted to snap a quick photo of us together. When I grabbed the phone to take a look, my belly looked distended. *I need to get into the nearest gym ASAP,* I thought.

We drove to the mall in Long Island to walk, shop, and talk like we used to back in undergrad. We got food from the food court, dropped the car off, and hailed a taxi back to the hotel. We sat on the balcony watching the Manhattan skyline and the pool party below in full force as the sun began to set. I said goodbye to my friend and her son and walked to the train station to catch the C train back home.

The train was delayed. As I waited in the cool evening air, my knees began to feel weak, and my breathing changed. I assumed I had had a long day running around the city and needed to rest. The train finally arrived and I immediately took the nearest seat by the doors. On the hour-long ride back to Brooklyn, I felt worse by the minute. My body was aching and I felt feverish. When I got home, I sat on the toilet, and this thing—whatever it was—was back.

A dark cloud enclosed me as I, for the 3rd month in a row, had the same symptoms and struggles. I started to put together and realize a pattern: this only happened during that time of the month. I was deeply concerned about the belly distension, the pain while going to the bathroom, my lack of appetite, and the nausea and exhaustion. Fear and dread began to cloud my thoughts. I scoured the Internet in search of a new gastroenterologist and found just the one.

I made an appointment to see Dr. Garrett in August. Upon our meeting, I immediately knew she was the one to help me. Dr. Garrett asked the golden question: "Crystal, what brings you in today? What's going on?" I told her what had happened over the last few months. She listened intently, requested blood work and another stool test, and told me to schedule an appointment with her office for a follow-up. If the blood work and stool test were inconclusive, she would suggest a complete colonoscopy. *A colonoscopy? It sounds like something people over 50 go through, not a 31 year old*, I thought.

Dr. Garrett called me a week later. My blood work results showed I had elevated inflammation markers but nothing alarming or abnormal. She called again within a few days and mentioned that the stool test had discovered the presence of blastocystis, but it is normal in adults and usually goes away on its own. Dr. Garrett suggested a medication that might help to resolve the blastocystis, but she was not confident it would resolve the issue. At this point, I was near desperation. I took the pills she prescribed, hoping the blastocystis was the culprit.

Dr. Garrett then suggested I consider a full colonoscopy in September, just to be thorough. I added it to my calendar. I trusted her.

Several days before my colonoscopy, I was tasked with prepping for the procedure. You are limited to certain foods for a few days, and you must ingest a bowel prep liquid solution that is far from tolerable for the average human. I knew things would be different for me as I had had some terrible drinks before—from herbal root drinks to shots of bad tequila. *This will not be hard to manage*, I thought, *I'm a tough little lady*. I mixed the liquid, stared at the solution, and began to chug it down. After a minute, I thought, *I knew I could do it—no big deal* and I got back to work.

Thirty seconds later, my stomach started to turn, and I began to salivate. I raced to the bathroom and barely made it to the toilet before I projectile vomited all of the liquid, while attempting to keep some down because this colonoscopy might be the answer to my questions. After cleaning the toilet, wiping my face, and brushing my teeth, I took a long look at myself in the mirror. I had to do this again this evening before bed; I also could not eat anything for the next 12 hours. Lovely.

The next day, Allen and I went to downtown Manhattan where the procedure would be performed. I paid the outrageous fee and sat in the waiting room until my name was called. Luckily, I had insurance and a free HSA account through my company. I whispered to Allen, "Can you believe how much they're charging for this? What if I didn't have any money?" We shook our heads. Within minutes, my name was called. I hugged Allen. "Don't worry," he said, "I'll see you soon."

As I walked with the nurse, she explained the numerous prep steps before leaving me to change into a robe with the back open and lay on a cold examination table. The anesthesia team started my IV, explained what would happen, and left as quickly as they had entered. Alone, I stared at my first IV. It hurt, but I was now used to pain. The surgery prep team came to get me moments later to take me back into the OR. I said a prayer, sighed, then all went dark.

I woke up to find water and crackers being shoved into my hands... I fell asleep and heard Allen gently waking me... Dr. Garrett entered and said I didn't get an A+ on my bowel prep. My system was not clear, so she couldn't perform a full colonoscopy. However, she had found a spot and decided to biopsy and send it to a lab; she said she would get in touch with me soon with a full update. I drifted back off to sleep for a moment. When I opened my eyes again, Allen was there with my clothes. Still under the pressure of the anesthetics, I dressed as fast as possible. The nurse came in, told me I was free to go, and went over discharge paperwork with me. Allen held me up with his forearm as I limped from the building and into the fresh chilled air. My body felt withered and frail as I hobbled, tired and drowsy from the meds.

One of my favorite lunch spots was near the train entrance. Allen ordered for us as I waited with my eyes closed. I was so glad it was over. I went home, showered, nibbled my food, and passed out until the next day.

A few days later, Dr. Garrett called: "Crystal, there is a large tumor in your rectum," she said, "I don't believe it's cancerous, but I need to confirm. I will alert you as soon as I hear back from the pathologist."

I didn't know what to think or how to feel. I waited.

After what felt like an eternity, Dr. Garrett called a few days later to confirm that I did not have colon cancer. *Thank God.* She asked if the symptoms were persisting around the time of my monthly cycle. I said yes. She then mentioned that although she was waiting for the full pathology report, the tissue was different and had traces of endometrial tissue. I then did the first thing most of us would do: I google searched "endometrial tissue" and soon learned a lot more on the subject than I could have imagined.

Dr. Garrett checked in a few days later to reconfirm: the tissue in the tumor was endometrial. Then her voice changed. She urgently recommended that I see a gynecologist ASAP. "Crystal," she said, "please keep in touch and provide me with updates on your symptoms and progress. If you need any referrals, I can assist." In a trembling voice, I give her warm regards and thanked her for supporting me over the past two months. My eyes began to water and blur; I knew that without her I would still be clueless. I ended the call just before the river of tears emerged.

Deep down, I could tell something was severely wrong. My world was suddenly crumbling right before my eyes. That night, I stayed up into the wee hours of the morning searching for a doctor and crying. I felt incomplete, lost—out of control. I'd never known what it meant to be sick. I'd had a cold a few times, but that was about it. The only time I'd ever been under a sedative was when I had decided my wisdom teeth needed to go because they crowded my teeth. Now this new word, *endometriosis*, was potentially impacting me. I was once invincible; now, I wasn't. I was once optimistic; now, I was unsure. I was once bold and courageous; now, I was weak and vulnerable.

After hours of reading, I remembered hearing about a doctor in my neighborhood having a specialty in endometriosis. I booked the first available appointment in October with Dr. Manor. I read at least 100 reviews and scoured the website to soak up as much knowledge about endometriosis as I could before drifting off to sleep with tears on my pillow.

2

BLINDSIDED

Let me rewind and explain a few things to you about my journey. I had the same gynecologist, Dr. Thompson, since I was 19 years old. Her bedside manner was unmatched and she genuinely cared for her patients. She recommended birth control for the painful periods, heavy bleeding, and acne. In college, my girlfriends and I referred to the pill as a tic tac. We'd say to one another, "Did you take your tic tac today?" I remember taking the pill for the more superficial reasons marketed to me by my doctor. It was an easy way to keep my skin clear because it kept hormones "in check" and was an easy way to know when my period would start and stop. The pill was a handicap. A cure-all. A mask over my reproductive organs to hide everything that was happening within.

I recall alerting Dr. Thompson a few years prior that I had been having excruciating cramps, more painful than usual. She'd told me I was on the strongest birth control available, but she could prescribe two pills for me, and I would need to take both to potentially get relief, but the side effects might be nasty. I had asked her to prescribe them and allow me to consider it. I didn't

take the second pill because I had been uncomfortable with the idea of taking
two birth control pills for cramps. Something hadn't seemed quite right about
that. I decided to continue my Aleve regimen and take one the day before my
cycle, two the morning of, and one or two every 6-12 hours from there. Over
time I came to know that, when that time of the month was coming, to brace
for impact and to stock up on supplies to get through it. We're taught that
pain is a normal part of becoming a woman. It's not.

On my 30th birthday, I traveled from New York to Alabama for my routine GYN visit. I also used the time to catch up with one of my best friends.
The Alabama air was refreshing, and the lack of sirens and cacophony,
soothing.

I pulled into the parking garage at Dr. Thompson's office, signed in, waited a few minutes, and walked back to meet with the nurse. I sat on the exam
table and waited for the doctor.

My routine had been unchanged for ten years. Dr. Thompson came in
with her usual radiant energy and asked if I had been checking my breasts
monthly. (Her recommended trick for remembering was for me to check my
breasts for abnormalities whenever I started a new birth control pill pack.)
She proceeded to perform my pap and pelvic exam, then commented that my
uterus seemed enlarged and I should have an ultrasound in the office to check
for fibroids. Well, that was new. I did know that there was a history of fibroids
on my maternal side. My mother, aunt, and grandmother had had fibroids
before they eventually felt forced into hysterectomies due to the lack of treatment options. My mother had been in her late forties when she had decided

to have a hysterectomy to rid herself of the trouble associated with fibroids. For some reason, I felt young and invincible and didn't think fibroids could happen to me.

I went into a small, dark room for an intravaginal ultrasound, a room I had always envisioned being in one day for a pregnancy checkup—not for this. But there I was. I waited for the doctor in her office. She confirmed I had fibroids. Three of them. I blamed the fibroids on my stressful career and decided some zen would fix it. I didn't need to worry—or so I assumed.

I spent the weekend in my hometown. Unbeknownst to me, Allen and my mom, along with my friends, had planned a birthday dinner for me. I was surprised and happy to see some of my favorite people in one room together. I enjoyed the moments with family and close friends and flew back to New York ready for the next adventure.

The following year, on my 31st birthday, I flew down again to see Dr. Thompson. This time, things were different: her tone had changed and she was no longer the doctor mom who gave hugs and exuded calmness in every uttered word. In a concerned tone, she said, "Crystal, your uterus has grown more, and so have the fibroids. You should get them removed as soon as possible."

I asked what the impacts were on conceiving. "Allen and I were talking about having children in the next few years."

"You should stop taking the birth control pills and try right away, but if you wait six months and come back to me, I would highly recommend surgery to remove the fibroids first."

My thirties were really beginning to be a nuisance. The news forced me to grow up. I felt like I was once a naive twenty-year-old college student and now a married woman with a demanding career and new health challenges. When I married, I vividly recall being unable to shake the thought of putting down the pill. I had been afraid of what would happen to my body without it and feared what I would look and feel like.

I heard a small voice inside telling me to stop taking the pill. I listened to that inner voice and thought this would be a good experience and a new chapter. During the first month off the pill, I noticed subtle changes, like oily skin, but nothing alarming—until the colonoscopy revealed what had been dormant in my body all these years... growing, spreading, increasing.

One chilly morning in October 2018, I sat in Dr. Manor's office in Brooklyn waiting to discuss the gastroenterologist's colonoscopy results. I held the printed copy in my hand and stared at it, my sweaty palms wrinkling the edges: I had a tumor, and based on my Internet reading, I likely had stage 4 deep infiltrating endometriosis. I took deep breaths to calm myself and patiently waited to be seen. Across from me were an expecting mother and another woman waiting for her sample birth control.

My name was finally called. I entered Room #2. I heard the doctor speaking jovially to another patient in an adjacent exam room.

After a short wait, Dr. Manor and a resident came in. Dr. Manor projected confidence as he sat, crossed his legs, and asked, "What's going on, Crystal?" I handed him my records, which he reviewed thoroughly with me. "Was endometriosis confirmed during the colonoscopy?" he asked.

"The pathologist suggested endometrial tissue but wasn't able to confirm it."

The doctor listened attentively. "Do you have plans to have children?"

"Yeah...yes I do."

He looked up. "Okay, here is what we need to do." He gave me a six-step action plan:

1. Pelvic Exam

2. Rectal Exam

3. Blood work

4. Ultrasounds (intra-vaginal and external)

5. CT scan

6. Laparoscopic Surgery (*Wait, what?*)

7. IVF referral, if needed

I tried to hold back tears in front of the doctor and his resident. I left the examination room replaying all the steps in my head until I'd memorized them.

I rolled up my sleeve for the nurse, to receive the first of many pricks in my arm. She was the nicest person in the office and made small talk about the weather. New York can be a tough place, so I appreciated her warmth as my mind drifted far into unknown territory. Next, I walked into a dark room labeled **Sonogram** and proceed to get photos taken of my insides. While undergoing the blood work and sonograms in the office that day, I realized I had a new task ahead of me, and I no longer felt sad: I felt ready to tackle this head-on and get it over with so I could move on with life. *Don't quit. You can handle this*, I told myself. I proceeded to get on the books for the CT scan and subsequently on the doctor's calendar for laparoscopic surgery. I set the date for November 8, 2018, and was sent on my way. As I left the office, I felt as if something had been stolen from me. I had done all the right things all those years, and hadn't known what was lying dormant in my body.

I walked back to my apartment in the bitter chill of late fall. I didn't care how cold it was; I wanted to sit for a bit. I found a place to sit and called Allen to tell him the news. His voice was somber but supportive. "You'll get through this," he said. I got home and began to research laparoscopic surgeries and what they entail. Then I decided the intelligent thing to do was get a second opinion, so I made an appointment with an OBGYN in Manhattan who seemed credible. By then, I had many questions about my reproductive health.

A week later, I took the train into the city, to the OBGYN's office for the second opinion. I spent approximately 10 minutes max in the room with her. She was perky and attentive. I asked if she could do an ultrasound of my fibroids and if she believed, based on my records, that this new diagnosis would impede pregnancy. She told me she outsources them to a nearby facility so she would be unable to do one and, based on my medical records, the fibroid seemed large but wouldn't impede a healthy pregnancy. She wrapped up by saying, "Come back and see me when you're pregnant," and waltzed out the room. That visit cost me $300 bucks. I'm still a bit salty about it, but I'm the one to blame: I was desperate for answers and knowledge, desperate to understand why the responses varied by doctor, and lost because there was not much awareness about the signs and symptoms of endo. I began to prepare myself for the reality of the eminent surgery.

Each month, the pain stayed longer than the previous month, and my exhaustion deepened due to the endo flares. I was implementing arguably the biggest project of my career thus far and training for the New York City Marathon, which was two days before my scheduled laparoscopic surgery with Dr. Manor.

In January, a friend and fellow mentor had convinced me to enter the lottery for the NYC Marathon because of my love for running. I was stunned when I checked my email one night in February and realized I'd won the lottery! So, I was going to race in one of the biggest marathons in the world. I was crushing it at work and training for the marathon in my spare time. Work was so busy, I didn't train as effectively as I could have. My mind was so preoccupied with endo, some days I didn't want to run but I did it anyway. One rainy Saturday morning, I did a few loops around Prospect Park and my bottom burned the entire run. I ran anyway. There was a war going on in my mind and I was constantly fighting. My mind wanted to quit, but I was determined not to let endo interfere with my dreams. *Life must go on*, I told myself.

It was now November. As usual, my cycle started around the beginning of the month. I was grateful for my remote work job: I could cover my belly in heat pads and blankets, and no one would ever know. I was killing it at work while the endo was attempting to kill me at home. Then Allen asked a question that had never occurred to me: "Are you sure you can go through with the marathon?" Truthfully, I was a wreck, but I told him I would finish the marathon, that dropping out was not an option. "Okay," he replied, as he gave me a hot blanket from the dryer to cover my distended belly. We had been married long enough that Allen knew the look in my eyes when I was determined to do something. However, I wholeheartedly understood why he had to ask the question. I was sitting at my desk with three heat pads on my pelvic area that I had bought from Duane Reade. I had used up almost all of the over-the-counter pain meds, but with endo, there is never enough heat, and rarely ever enough pain meds to relieve the symptoms.

My mom flew up to NYC the day before the marathon to cheer me on along my 26.2-mile journey and to support me after surgery. She had recently retired, so she could stay with me during recovery while Allen worked. By the way, the only race I had ever entered before was a 5K and that had been at least four years ago. I didn't perceive this as a challenge though—one of my primary mantras is mind over matter. We (human beings) are usually the ones in our own way. My parents divorced when I was two years old. My father was a Vietnam vet and had problems of his own. When they split, he left my mother a single mom with no financial support, plus all the joint bills to pay. My mom worked tirelessly around the clock and never complained. My strength and resiliency come from her, my grandparents, and my upbringing. We got through things. Ironically, my mom would soon watch my core and legs propel me to the finish, and two days later, she would watch me struggle to stand up on the same legs unassisted.

Marathon day was here. My cycle had come and gone. I was excited and I couldn't believe I was going to do this. I ate a light breakfast, stretched, meticulously put on my gear, said my goodbyes to Allen and Mom, popped in my air pods, and hit the elevator. After what felt like forever (two trains, one ferry, one bus, and a lot of walking), I stood with the other runners at the starting point on the Staten Island bridge. The energy was contagious. Everyone was looking out to the left, in awe of the view of the Manhattan skyline.

The countdown began as a mob of people travelled in unison over the bridge, slowly making their own pace. The sun beamed and the wind carried us forward. After each passing mile, my confidence grew. Around mile 15, I took a bathroom break. After what had happened in Bali, I was a tad cautious. I peed in the port-a-potty and, to my relief, everything was clear. Yes! I told my body to keep going and not quit. I memorized every positive sign I saw in the crowd of onlookers and allowed the messages to push me through the next mile. As I ran, I thought about my endo journey and how I planned to run again one day and wear a shirt that said, "I survived endo." I finished the marathon strong, coming in at around 5 hours and 20 minutes. For a first-time marathoner, I felt proud. For the first time in months, I was flying high without the trailing negative thoughts of endo. For 26.2 miles, my body did what my mind told it to do and that felt good. I was a finisher, not a quitter. I held these positive thoughts captive in preparation for what was to come.

3

✺

CATEGORY 4

November 8, 2018. I opened my eyes and took a deep breath; surgery day was finally here. Around 7a.m., my mom, Allen, and I walked to the surgery center, around 0.2 miles from my apartment. The receptionist checked my insurance policy and informed me that the center would bill me for the surgery, and that any checks I received from the insurance company should be forwarded to them. I waited with my family for about ten minutes before I was called to get dressed for surgery. I said my goodbyes to my mom and Allen and nervously walked to the dressing room with the nurse. She explained that I needed to take everything off, including anything with metal. I stripped down to nothing, removed the hair tie and pins from my hair, and placed the surgical cap on my head. I was then ushered to a cold, sterile sitting area with other surgery candidates—all with somber looks.

Eventually, I was taken to a curtained section of the room, where I sat in the cold hospital chair. Several nurses came to check my vitals and to prepare my IV. Then the anesthesiologist came. He began to chat in an Eastern European accent I could hardly understand. I hoped and trusted all would be well and nodded in agreement to receive the anesthesia. Dr. Manor came in eventually and explained what to expect and that this was an exploratory surgery meant to diagnose endo and he would excise any endo he could. I would have three incisions on my belly and receive discharge instructions when I woke from surgery.

The nurse assistant sat with me for a while, until a nurse retrieved me and said that Allen wanted to see me. I walked out and met his eyes, which were searching to make sure I was okay. I told him I hadn't been taken back to the operating room yet. Allen felt relieved to lay eyes on me. He kissed my forehead and said, "Everything will be okay." It didn't *feel* okay.

I walked back to the waiting area, and the nurse explained I needed to trash the gown and socks I had on and replace them with new clean ones. I had only stepped out for 10 seconds, but I was thankful for their thoroughness.

After an hour or two, the doctor came from the operating room to apologize for the delay and explained that he was dealing with a cancer patient, whom he had had to attend to. I was fine with this, as I would want someone to understand my situation too, albeit the difference.

I fell asleep waiting, until suddenly I was awakened and rushed to a massive operating room with intimidating equipment. There were two male nurses and the anesthesiologist. They said they would take good care of me and I won't feel a thing while under the knife. The anesthesiologist began counting down. All went black.

My vision went in and out as I fought to stay awake. I was in the recovery room and the nurse was handing me a cup of water. I drank some and spilled the rest on my gown as I faded out of consciousness again.

When I woke, the nurse told me I needed to go to the bathroom and urinate before I was released. *Good*, I thought, *I need to get out of here.* But, I struggled to move. My legs felt wobbly. It was difficult moving anything below my navel without having something to hold on to. The nurse allowed me to lean on her to get to the bathroom. Once there, she closed the door and I sat on the toilet trying not to fall to the floor. I peed and after getting up, I noticed dried blood on the toilet. I cleaned it the best I could and turned to wash my hands. Before I could finish, my stomach churned violently. With a hunched back, I hobbled dizzily over to the toilet, aiming vomit toward it. I cleaned up again and splashed water on my face. Barely standing, I managed to open the door and a nurse helped me to the changing room. In a stupor, I somehow got dressed.

The place was almost empty. I was alone. *I must have been in surgery for quite some time*, I thought to myself. I gripped the wall, looked for the exit, opened the door, and saw my mom—everyone else was gone. Unable to speak, I waved her over to help me stand.

"I need to get out of here," I said.

"Take it easy. Allen is trying to flag down a car ... it's raining really hard."

I was eager to crash on my bed. "No, I'm going to walk the two blocks."

With Allen on one side and my mother on the other, we walked home. Two days ago, I had averaged 10-11-mph splits; now, I could barely walk.

In the comfort of my home, I showered, brushed my teeth, and prepared for bed with my mother's help. She told me to rest and left the bedroom. Allen came in; he knew I would want all the details before I could sleep. He relayed that the surgery, which had been originally estimated to be one to two hours, had lasted five hours. The doctor had confirmed that deep infiltrating endometriosis was the issue and had removed the little he could. Because of how deep the endo was in my pelvic area, I would need a second surgery. Allen told me my mom, upon hearing the news, had been alarmed and shaken as this was her first time hearing, directly from the doctor, about the endo wrecking the body of her only child and only hope for grandchildren. The doctor had told them that the endo was stage 4 and that, unfortunately, most of it was located in and around the rectum. During the second go-around, he would need a second surgeon specializing in colon-related procedures: a colorectal surgeon. It looked as though my reproductive anatomy was distorted due to huge fibroids hanging off my uterus, and my tubes appeared blocked, but it could also be that the fibroids were smushing them.

Another surgery? That was too much to hear. I thanked Allen for being there for me. He kissed my forehead and I drifted off to sleep.

4

EYE OF THE STORM

Over the next two weeks, I could barely get out of bed without a cane or someone helping me up. Fortunately, my mom stayed with us for a week. She cooked the best southern food each night, determined to nurse me back to health with each meal. During my first week of recovery, the surgery center called to make sure all was well and told me I would need to make a two-week follow-up appointment with the doctor. After one week, my mom went home and I returned to work. It was not too bad since I didn't have to leave my home.

Two weeks post-surgery, with the temperature hovered over freezing in NYC, I walked over to my doctor's office feeling needle pricks with each step. The walk was symbolic of my endo path —painful and relentless.

My doctor explained that the pathology results were not back yet, but he could review his surgery notes with me, and we should plan for the next steps. He repeated what Allen had already relayed and showed me pictures of the lesions and a dark, disturbing area near my rectum that had been causing me debilitating pain throughout the month. He wanted me to have another surgery in roughly three months, and till then, start on a drug that had recently hit the market called Orilissa. Just months prior, the drug had not been available to consumers but had been recently approved. He said it was costly but worth it. He would have the receptionist call the local pharmacy, which his office worked with, and I would not have to pay. The drug would suppress the endo and keep the inflammation at bay until I was back on the operating table. *Reduced endo symptoms? Count me in!*

I left the office hopeful—but cautious. The wind stung and pushed me as I walked back home and mentally added this new drug to the checklist of things to do before I could live normally again. Would that ever happen? *Yes*, I thought, *stay positive.*

As Thanksgiving approached, I called the pharmacy every other day to check on the Orilissa. Each time, the pharmacy explained that the prior authorization from my doctor and insurance company hadn't gone through. I returned to the doctor's office to push them a bit. They explained they had sent everything off, but they would try a new (and tiny) pharmacy in Queens, the only other location in the NYC metro area with Orilissa on hand. My prescription was transferred there. Major pharmacies were not carrying the drug yet. I spoke to the pharmacist in Queens, who explained that prescriptions for Orilissa had been flooding the pharmacy since they were one of the few authorized to fill it. She explained I should keep her posted on any side effects and she would call me occasionally to check in.

Eventually, after two attempts, and once I explained to the pharmacy that I had had endo surgery and had taken birth control as a medication, the prior authorization was finally approved. Apparently, I had to have my stomach cut open, blown up, and had to take meds to get the insurance company's approval to get the new drug.

Gold in pill form was delivered to my home a few days later. I read the entire pamphlet with Allen before I took the little pink pill. I decided the potential results were worth the possible side effects—I wanted relief from my pain and suffering.

In January 2019, my symptoms were nearly gone except for the mucus in my stool. The Orilissa was working well. I felt better than I had in months. My cycle was light, almost nonexistent. The only noticeable change was my hair. Shortly after taking the pill, my hair had begun to shed like I'd never experienced before. Every time I ran my fingers through my hair, strands were left in my palm. I could tell it was shedding from the root and was not breakage. I would sit and stare at the strands in my hand. My hair was something I loved about myself. It was always shiny and full of body. The hair loss impacted my self-esteem, a lot. Now, I dreaded brushing it and I kept it pulled back in a ponytail. If I wore my hair otherwise, strands would fall onto my shoulders. I thought it was either short-term side effects of the anesthesia or a random side effect of the pink pill. I alerted the pharmacist when she called to check-in.

I spent December and January waiting on my next surgery so I could be done and start living life again. In the meantime, I'd changed my dietary lifestyle. I cut all processed foods and was vegan 9 meals out of 10. I was trying to do everything within my power to live a healthier lifestyle. I was learning how much food plays a role in how our endocrine systems function. The Orilissa was working, but my hair was growing thinner by the day, and the mucus in my stool, more prominent. No one knew the actual long-term effects of this stuff, but I was desperate. I would eventually need to make the call: either continue to lose hair or fall back into the pool of debilitating pain.

I took the Orilissa for about two months, then called it quits. I had a six-month prescription available, but I called the pharmacy and requested that they discontinue its delivery. It was a tough decision, but I knew deep down that if my hair was falling, it was potentially impacting my hormones in other ways unbeknownst to me.

In February 2019, after waiting patiently for my body to heal from surgery, I called Dr. Manor's office to inquire about scheduling my second laparoscopic surgery. I reached a curt, abrupt receptionist who acted as if I'd ruined her day by calling.

"Um, I would like to make an appointment to see the doctor and schedule my subsequent surgery," I said.

Her response knocked me off-kilter: "Dr. Manor is working from Miami for the remainder of the winter and only sees patients a few times per month on Mondays in New York City. There is no clear date on when he will be back and can perform surgeries."

I will say, that was one smart guy. NYC winters can be brutal, so that was a pretty genius idea. I hung up with the receptionist and proceeded to check the doctor's Instagram page. He was a quirky fellow and requested that his patients DM him on IG with any questions. The sun and palm trees looked delightful in the background and now he was specializing in vaginal reconstruction. He could have his fun in South Beach, but I was determined to have this surgery in the next two months. The pain level was starting to creep back up, and I wasn't sure if there was a cap to the pain I could experience with this disease stirring in the depths of my pelvis. *Now what?* I thought to myself. I scoured the Internet for a new doctor, again.

I had lived in NYC for three years and I didn't really have a GYN there, so I decided to research the best doctors and surgeons specializing in endo instead. I immediately got a list of hits on Yelp. I searched their websites and watched video testimonials. I had no idea some clinics and doctors specialized only in endo. This was eye-opening for me. I spent hours reading reviews and stories from women all over the globe who travelled to visit these doctors. The next day, I decided to call the 1st and 2nd highest ranking doctors to find how soon I could get an appointment. I submitted an online inquiry for #1 and #2. I assumed that for #1 on the list, the wait for surgery would be far too long, so I called #2 first hoping to get lucky. The receptionist at #2 mentioned it may be several months before I could have surgery. *Um, no. I need surgery today.* I called #1. The heavens opened. The friendly receptionist answered the phone. Over the next 10 minutes, I felt as though my soul had become at peace—someone understood what I was going through and that I urgently needed to be seen. The angel on the other end of the phone explained the process and the cost of the first consultation. She told me I was a perfect candidate for their offices and that they looked forward to helping me. The office did not accept insurance and was out of network. I didn't blink an eye about the price because I needed help—badly. There went that desperation again and more money out of the door. My appointment was set for March 10th at 10a.m.

Over the next month, I struggled to keep social engagements. At this point, the Orilissa should have been out of my system. My hair stopped shedding excessively, but the endo symptoms returned with full force. In early March, for the first time, there was a speckle of blood in the mucus. It was a clear sign I was not well. I could hear my heart beating in my ears. Over the last few months, going to the bathroom around my cycle had become difficult. I would lose half of my energy reserves. It was excruciating, *every time*. It felt as though my body was caving in on me, but I kept going.

On March 10ᵗʰ, Allen and I arrived at the doctor's office on the Upper East Side, earlier than my appointment. There were fresh flowers, marble countertops, and cozy, inviting seats in the waiting area. I signed in, and the receptionists were real-life angels there to guide me to the promised land. I waited nervously, patiently. There was a woman with a suitcase, as if she had flown in to see the doctors. All of us looked different—different ethnicities and religions—but we were all there because of something that had chosen us.

I'd brought my records from my gastroenterologist who had discovered the endometrial tissue, and documents from the first surgery in Brooklyn.

I was soon called back to meet with Dr. Glover. I had read on the site that she had had five laparoscopic surgeries for endo and specialized in it; she had understanding due to her own journey. Dr. Glover was warm, beautiful, refreshing, and she carried a maternal air. I felt safe. Dr. Glover reviewed my records, asking questions along the way. When I told her my story, she was empathetic and explained what was happening to me as though she was reading my mind: she made assumptions about my symptoms that were 100% accurate. She explained that they would need to perform an ultrasound to get a better look with a 3D imaging machine for better visibility.

I went into the ultrasound room, removed my bottoms, and covered myself with the gown. Dr. Glover returned with Dr. Samil, the surgeon who had established this practice. They looked at my uterus, measured the fibroids, and told me they could take them out with no problem. They captured many photos, then asked me to get dressed and come into a third room to review my case and next steps.

I dressed and walked into a room with a super high-tech screen on the wall. The doctors explained the surgery would be extensive and that they would need a colorectal surgeon. They would need to remove the fibroids, check my tubes, excise the endo, and remove the endo tumor from my rectum. They drew an image on the board and showed me exactly what would happen during the surgery. I now knew I was in the right place, and I was eager to schedule the surgery. "How soon can I have the surgery?" I asked. They explained I would need to get a full MRI so they could have the clearest image possible prior to surgery. I would also need to return to the office twice before surgery: one visit to review the MRI results and one pre-op visit a day or two before the operation. *More steps*, I thought. I shook hands with the surgeons and I told them I was ready to be reborn. I headed back to the front desk to schedule my follow-up with the receptionist and pay the fees. She gave me the prescription and instructions for scheduling the MRI. I felt so relieved, and Allen and I chatted about the next steps all the way back to Brooklyn.

On March 13th, I finished work and jumped on the train to the Upper East Side for my MRI appointment in the evening. The nurse explained I should undress and take off any metal; she needed to start an IV in my arm and would give me headphones for the duration of the MRI. *One step closer.* I was willing to do whatever it took to get this surgery scheduled.

I asked the receptionist when to expect the results. She said they would be sent to the doctor's office within one business day, and I would receive the results in the mail in about one week. Great. I wasn't thrilled about the out-of-network prices, but the service was worth it. The next day, I called to schedule my follow-up with the surgeons. I was set for March 22nd.

The MRI results came back, and it was a detailed, ugly reminder of how bad my situation was. The tumor was sitting near the S3 sacral nerve.

March 22nd came. I met with Dr. Le in the office. Dr. Le was one of three surgeons in the practice. She reviewed my file, updated the office notes with details from the MRI, and answered all my questions about what to expect without hesitation. She mentioned that they typically worked with a few colorectal surgeons and recommended that I meet with the colorectal surgeon and ask questions before the surgery. I would also need a primary care physician to perform a pre-op clearance, including a physical, EKG, and blood work before the operation. As I took in this news, I started to plan when I could squeeze the visits into my busy work schedule. I was so close to surgery though, I could taste it. The receptionist explained that there was a slot around the end of April for surgery, but she would need to confirm the dates with the colorectal surgeon and get back to me. She said Dr. Ari appeared to be free, but she would need to double-check. She suggested that I make an appointment with him to discuss my case before returning.

When I got home, I booked an appointment for April 8th with Dr. Ari and searched for a primary care physician. I hadn't had one since I was 17 years old. I set up another appointment to meet with a nurse practitioner on the Upper West Side to perform my pre-op clearance work for April 22nd. A few days later, the angel posed as a receptionist contacted me to explain that the earliest I could get in for surgery was April 26th, and she would confirm with the colorectal surgeon. I held my breath and prayed that the schedules would align. The receptionist reached out the next day and said I would have the surgery in exactly one month. April 26th was the date. *Yes, yes, yes!* Finally, I was close.

April arrived. At that point, I was traveling to Pittsburgh every week for work. For the fourth time over the last few weeks, I had canceled dinner plans with colleagues due to my debilitating pain. I couldn't sleep. I could barely move. My stomach was distended roughly 5 inches, but I hid it well. My 32nd birthday was in a few days; however, celebrating was the furthest thing from my mind.

I woke on April 2nd and took a picture of my belly. The right side of my stomach was higher than the left. *Was this endo or the massive fibroid?* Exhausted from lack of sleep, I took painstaking steps to my suitcase to find medicine and realized I was running low. I needed a new supply to get through the workday, so I dressed in casual clothes and mapped out the nearest pharmacy. I walked through a light mist of rain to the nearest location (a longer walk than I would have liked), bought more meds, and paid the outrageous price for heat pads. I needed at least two heat pads on my abdomen and pelvis, one wrapped around my back, and one hot hands pack for an extra layer of heat between my pants and underwear. The throbbing, relentless pain I couldn't alleviate was in my rectum; it felt as if my insides would spill and expose my innermost parts.

I didn't look the same. I didn't feel the same.

I counted down the days in my head: *24*—and my cycle hadn't started yet.

Gingerly, I returned to the hotel to get dressed. I slowly peeled back the adhesive, added the heat pads, took the pain meds, and ate a granola bar before taking the elevator down to the lobby where I would meet my coworker, pretending I was perfectly fine.

On April 4th, I landed in NYC and took a taxi home. After managing a few half smiles at the front desk staff, I slid into the elevator and rode up to our apartment gripping the elevator rails so hard my hands hurt. I hobbled to the bathroom, barely speaking to Allen, though I had been out of town for four days. I was nauseous and my bowels were bloated—angry. A pool of blood poured into the toilet bowl. Tears welled in my eyes as my body convulsed in unspeakable pain. The groans and howls from the bathroom brought a fearful look to Allen's face. I shut the bathroom door shaking, mascara running.

"Are you okay?" Allen yelled.

No, no, no, I am not okay.

I opened the bathroom door and crawled toward the bed, sweating and squirming—my breathing, labored. My cycle was not here. What was happening? On all fours, I crawled back to the bathroom in agony, then I realized ... the tumor had breached my rectum and eroded the remaining rectal wall separating the endometrial tumor from my bowels. The tumor was bleeding and now blocking my rectum. Trying to excrete with DIE (Deep Infiltrating Endometriosis) feels like the acronym suggests: DEATH. After sitting on the toilet, my energy reserves were depleted, I nearly fainted. My body began to shake as more blood seeped into the toilet. I placed tissue in my undies and began to pray on the hard, cold floor. I wailed in agony; in deep lament. *I will live and not die. I will live and not die. I will not die*, I whispered to myself.

Allen was worried. "We need to call the doctors! What if you need emergency surgery?"

"No... It's late," I cried, "I'll try to tough it out."

It wasn't long before Allen went against my wishes and called the doctor's office. The on-call service picked up and the representative said the doctor on call would phone shortly. It was about 1 a.m. I lay on the floor, on my stomach, covered with only a blanket, panties and bra on, squirming, moving in and out of consciousness. Dr. Le called, and in a terrified but firm voice, I told her that blood was coming from my rectum in a way it hadn't before. Sleepily, she said, "I want you to go to the Lenox Hill emergency room and have a CT scan done first thing in the morning. We need to ensure there isn't a total blockage in the rectum." In my mind, a blockage equated to emergency surgery and I didn't feel this was the case. Allen told Dr. Le he had given me one Tylenol with Codeine pill, from the November surgery, for the pain. Dr. Le advised me to begin taking meds every three hours and said I needed to keep something in my system for the pain, mainly for the inflammation, then we ended the call. Allen walked to the nearest store to get some meds for me.

I took two tablets of Tylenol Extra Strength 500mg. Three hours later, I took three tablets of Ibuprofen 200mg per tab. An hour later, Dr. Le called back, this time wide awake. She had reviewed my file more and decided we should cancel the emergency room visit; she thought I was experiencing period symptoms. I was shocked that she thought this because whatever this was felt completely unrelated—but I trusted her.

Allen helped me to the bed and I slipped under the covers. Somehow, while moving in and out of consciousness and maybe getting one hour of sleep, I woke to see another day, and my cycle did appear, just as the heavenly expert had expected.

On April 5th, Allen decided to work from home and run errands for me during lunch. I asked him to bring back more of the meds Dr. Le had suggested and some Depends. *Depends—that was where I was in life.* In one day, I would be a 32-year-old woman needing Depends diapers. It hit me that I was having two periods: blood was pouring from two places, and pads weren't designed to handle that. Every conceivable question about my life came to mind: *How was this possible? Why me? What had I did wrong? I thought God loved me, but does he still?* What if I had been born in 1800? I would have died from this. My death would have been imminent. That thought depressed me more than anything.

When Allen returned with pills and Depends, I showered, changed, took the pills, and slipped back into bed with tears falling from my eyes. I alternated between crying and sleeping. I had no appetite. No desire for life. My social life was nonexistent: no social media posts or dinner dates with the girls. I got up and worked as much as I could, and after 5:30p.m., I logged out and slowly made my way back to bed. I received a few Happy Birthday text messages and calls, but scared I may burst into tears, I couldn't bring myself to respond or answer the phone. What I feared most was anyone feeling sorry for me.

Allen tried to cheer me up. "I have a surprise for your birthday tomorrow," he said, "if you're up for it. I got tickets to the Hamilton Broadway show and reservations at a Chinese restaurant in Chinatown after. A few weeks back, I purchased insurance on the tickets just in case you weren't feeling well." I perked up and told him I was going to the show even if I had to crawl into the theatre. He smiled. "That's my girl."

April 6th—the day I was born and another year around the sun. My face was pale; I didn't look well. Somehow, I managed to get dressed to see the show in Manhattan, which was fantastic. I felt an overwhelming gratitude for my partner, for his patience and helpfulness with my sad mood. For the first time in my life, I was depressed. I didn't want to see or speak to anyone. Sitting through Hamilton had exhausted the energy I had had to get through the rest of the day. My bottom burned as every burst of rectal blood stole my reserves and my birthday. We didn't make it to Chinatown for dinner, but we went home, ordered takeout, and watched a movie. I fell asleep on the couch. Cheers to 32.

On the morning of April 8th, I took the train to Midtown Manhattan to meet with Dr. Ari, the colorectal surgeon. I signed in, sat, and waited. After a few minutes, my name was called and I was greeted by the assistant, whom I followed to the examination room. She told me to wait. A minute later, Dr. Ari walked in. His demeanor was calm and kind as he asked me about my history. I shared my story, which was, sadly, getting longer. I told him about the previous surgery and how the gastroenterologist had discovered the issue. He asked about my symptoms. I told him the wound was getting deeper, and about the rectal pain. He asked me if I had seen blood in the stool. I told him about what had happened last week and the pain med regimen I was currently on. Several questions later, he told me he wanted to examine my abdomen and perform a rectal exam. I winced. Embarrassed, I told him I was on my cycle and bleeding from the rectum, so I had a Depends on. He was unphased. He'd seen it all, I supposed.

I climbed onto the exam table and the doctor returned with the assistant. He pushed and pressed on each of the four abdominal quadrants, and then I turned to my side so he could check my rectum. Holding in a scream, I gritted my teeth and squeezed the exam table until my knuckles grew pale. The doctor popped off the gloves and remarked, "The rectal examination seems consistent with the MRI results. There is a tumor and it feels like it is pushing out from the wall of the rectum and impacting a significant portion. It's quickly beginning to create a blockage in the colon. Sometimes we can shave out the tumor from the rectum but, in this case, it would be a highly unlikely option. In your case, it's a high likelihood we will have to remove that part of the rectum and reconnect the ends. If I can shave it, I will, because it's a more straightforward procedure. If I believe the hole left behind would be too large, though, you will need an anterior resection of the rectum. I will decide in the operating room. We will try to do it laparoscopically. We may have to make an incision to get that part of the rectum out of the body. There are risks of the operation: bleeding and infection. The main issue is the connection. When reconnected, there is a slight chance of failure. If something goes wrong, you could get very sick and need to be rushed to the hospital to save your life."

My mind drifted. I was sure I had just heard that if anything went wrong, I could die. I regained composure and pulled out my list of questions. "How long should I plan to be in the hospital?"

"About 4-5 days. Recovery will be slow. I will probably have to remove 50% or more of the rectum based on the examination and MRI results. There is a tiny percentage of a small hole in the connection that would cause leakage. If this occurs, it could potentially impact your fertility. I will perform an ileostomy if there is a chance of leakage. An ileostomy is a bag that hangs from your belly and allows your intestines to empty the feces without going through the bowels. Now, even with surgery, endometriosis can come back. We should get you feeling better, but it could last a few months, a few years, or a lifetime. The resection is riskier, but the long-term effects may be worth it. You will need antibiotics a day before the surgery and a bowel prep kit to clean the body. You should fast 12 hours before the surgery and not eat or drink anything."

I left the doctor's office, forcing back tears. (I walked around with sunglasses on because crying was now a daily thing.) I moved into the thick smoggy air of NYC and reflected on everything I had just heard, not sure what to say or think. The surgery I'd been waiting on for months could potentially kill me. There are always standard risks associated with surgery, but for some reason, the stakes this time seemed more tangible. If I didn't get the tumor removed, I could die. If I *did* get the tumor removed, I could die. I didn't feel I had a choice. But, despite feeling depressed, I chose life.

I planned to take two weeks off work. I had life insurance through my company and not much debt, but I felt the need to take out a policy just in case the worst happened. But, guess what? If you have been to the doctor as much as I had in the past year, the insurance companies will deny you a decent policy, which brought me to tears again. The emotional toll meant many sleepless nights, along with the physical pain. I faced the days ahead in agony.

On April 22nd, I took the 2 train uptown to see a nurse practitioner to complete my pre-surgery requirements. The NP was young and helpful. She explained I would need to provide blood for vials, a urine sample, and an EKG to ensure I was healthy enough for the surgery (ironic, I think). She explained that the lab usually takes a few days to process the blood, but she should be able to rush it and clear me in time.

By the evening of April 23rd, I received a portal notification from the NP stating that everything had come back normal, and I should be clear to proceed with surgery on Friday. She faxed the paperwork over to the surgeon's office, so I was good to go. She noted that my CA-125 levels were incredibly high, which could be from the endometriosis, but said I should have the surgeons confirm. I internet searched "CA-125" after the call. It stands for Cancer Antigen 125 and is used to measure signs of ovarian cancer and other cancers. *My God.* More tears erupted. *What else could possibly go wrong?* It was now less than 48 hours before my surgery.

On April 24th, I went uptown for my pre-op work at the surgeon's office. I waited nervously. The nurse emerged from the back, "Crystal? Come with me." I provided a urine sample, then went to the ultrasound room. I urinated, undressed for the ultrasound, and waited with my legs in stirrups.

"How are you feeling?" the nurse asked, "Nervous? Excited? Can't believe it's already here?"

"It's my second birthday," I replied, "A chance at a new start."

She smiled. "Well, Happy Birthday... The doctor will be right in."

Dr. Le entered with Dr. Samil, the practice's head GYN surgeon, by her side and immediately dimmed the lights. They reviewed my chart and records.

"How are you doing?" Dr. Samil asked.

"Okay."

Dr. Le said, "You are the first case on Friday morning."

Dr. Samil asked her, "What are we doing on Friday?"

"Myomectomy, excision, bowel resection."

"What is the second case we're doing on Friday?"

"Excision only."

I interpreted that to mean that there were only two cases or patients in surgery on Friday: me and another woman whom I did not know but felt sorry for. Dr. Le then told him, "Crystal's is slotted for four hours." Dr. Samil then proceeded to comment on how huge my fibroids are, which I had heard more times than I would have liked. "How old are you?"

"32."

Dr. Samil stared at the screen and took some pictures. He then explained that there would be a small C-section-like incision on my abdomen due to the bowel resection and the rest will be tiny incisions. I was told to go ahead and get dressed and meet him back in his office for the last touchpoint before Friday.

In the office, Dr. Samil reviewed my thick chart once more and asked when and if I had met with the colorectal surgeon. "Two weeks ago." He continued to plow through my file with his glasses on his nose—such a peculiar and brilliant man with mad scientist-like movements—his brain constantly processing information. I was grateful he was that way. After he finished reading, he said, "We're all set. We will remove all the fibroids and you should be okay."

I needed to be at the hospital at 6:30a.m, so I confirmed the address and location to quell any doubts about where I was going on Friday. "Doctor, what should I anticipate for recovery time?" I asked.

"Three to four days in the hospital and six weeks from surgery. No travel for at least four weeks. Let's see how it goes, but don't plan anything." He walked me out and I confirmed Allen would be with me on Friday. After the doctor left, the receptionist told me the details for Friday. She was kind, serious and efficient. *Be there at 6:30am. Go to Lenox Hill. Check in. Head to the 10th floor.* The receptionist then pulled me into one of the doctors' offices for privacy and explained the process for reserving a hospital room and the costs affiliated with a private versus semi-private room. The hospital's protocol would be to call me and ask about these details and I could confirm my requests at that time. I was completely overwhelmed but also excited. Reality was beginning to set in. After Friday, my life would be forever changed.

Winter was leaving NYC and the sun was out. I jumped in an Uber and headed home to continue the workday.

Everyone at the office was aware that I was having surgery, but no one knew it was life threatening.

5

JOY IN THE MORNING

pril 25th. 8:30a.m. I worked feverously to ensure my teams were prepared to move and operate without me. At the same time, my mind was occupied with the pre-surgery prep required by both the gynecological and colorectal surgeons to be deemed ready to proceed. This was the combined schedule:

12p.m. — Cytotec (1 pill)

3p.m. — Metronidazole (1 pill)

3p.m. — Neomycin (2 pills)

4p.m. — Prepopik powder

7p.m. — Neomycin (2 pills)

11p.m. — Prepopik powder

11p.m. — Metronidazole (1 pill)

12a.m. — Shower with Hibiclens

12a.m. — No food or drinks

I didn't know what all the pills were for, but I chugged them down at the appropriate timeslots. The prepopik powder only stayed down briefly—I vomited. I'd been there before, in preparation for my colonoscopy, but this time I realized I should just succumb to the idea that I would be sick from 4p.m. until 2a.m.

Around 6p.m., I got ready for movie night and the last date night I would have in a while. I had purchased tickets to the *Avengers: End Game* premiere at the Regal UA on Court Street. It was the first showing of the night and tickets had been sold out for weeks. A month ago, I had remembered that the movie would premiere on Friday, April 26th, the same day as my surgery. To Allen's surprise, I had sat in an online waiting room to buy the tickets the day they had opened for purchase and, luckily, they were showing in NYC one night earlier. I threw on jeans, a cute shirt, my favorite leather jacket, and booties. At 7p.m., I took the two pills of Neomycin with water and I was out the door. I walked over to the theatre, enjoying the evening air.

Allen arrived from work just in time for us to walk around the crowds and straight into the movie theatre. Watching the film, I felt mixed emotions. I was happy to be out enjoying my final day of freedom and mobility for the next two weeks, but I was also naturally concerned about what the next day had in store. I made it through the movie and held back my tears and fears.

Three hours later, we left the movie theatre hand-in-hand and hopped in a taxi for the 10-block ride home. During the ride, reality started to set in, and tears began to stream down my cheeks. Though I had tried my hardest to be tough and control them, they kept coming. My journey to my own endgame was just beginning.

Around 11p.m., I take my next round of meds and prep. I continued fi-
nalizing instructions for my coworkers and sending out any last emails. Between vomiting and diarrhea from the powder, I managed to submit all as-
signments and instructions around midnight. Officially relieved, I could then
focus solely on my health for the next week or so. I moved from the couch
to the toilet an uncountable number of times. Allen was fast asleep and I felt
anger well up inside me. I wasn't upset with Allen but upset about the turn
of events in my life. It felt unfair. I washed my hands the millionth time and
checked my hospital bag once more to be sure I had everything I needed. I
prayed and cried again until I finally fell asleep around three in the morning.

6

HAPPY RE-BIRTH DAY

April 26. The day I'd awaited for far too long was finally here. I woke around 5a.m., fatigued, with blood-red eyes. I told myself I would get plenty of sleep under anesthesia and sitting in the hospital. Allen woke and gave me a hug. I slipped on tights and my sweatshirt from the New York City Marathon I had completed just six months ago.

Allen's uncle, Ray, had a brand-new Tesla and offered to drive me to the hospital. I was relieved by this simple gesture. On the ride up to Lenox Hill Hospital, there was small talk about the car and current events. Uncle Ray asked if I was ready and said to not be nervous. I told him I was ready to get it over with and move on with my life. As we approached the hospital, a glimmer of light hit the high rises and skyscrapers in select places.

Uncle Ray dropped us off, gave me a hug, and told Allen that if he found a parking space, he would come in to sit with us for a while. We entered the hospital, showed ID, got our pictures taken, and I let the admissions receptionists know I was there for surgery on the 10th floor. They pointed us in the direction of the registration area directly across the hall. I took my paperwork and waited in line to sign in. I was told what the upfront fees were and was given a stack of papers to fill out. After tons of signatures and initials, I returned the documents and paid the hospital fees. The woman at the front desk called someone upstairs to confirm my surgery date and time and told them she was sending me up. I thanked her, then Allen, Uncle Ray, and I headed upstairs. The woman on the 10th floor was your typical New Yorker. In a loud, direct, raspy voice that seemed endearing to me in the moment, she told me I needed to leave all valuables with a family member. She would be taking me to the back soon. I signed another set of documents and started to grow nervous. After a few encouraging words from Allen and Uncle Ray, I nodded. This was just the next stop on my train. I was ready for a new start, I took a deep breath. Seconds later, the petite, feisty, raspy-voiced woman walked toward me. She pointed to a door that was one way in, by badge access only. I had only two seconds to wave goodbye to my family before I followed the woman through the doors of no return.

Inside, I was greeted by a bustling pre-op area filled with humans and their loved ones sitting nearby in 6x6 areas cornered off by sheets that are being whipped around like shower curtains. A nurse swiftly approached and took me to my own 6x6 area to begin changing from regular clothes into a hospital gown. She told me I needed a urine sample and to empty my bladder. No problem. I had had an overactive bladder for years, thanks to the fibroids. I walked into the bathroom and used the little plastic cup to provide a urine sample and I emptied my bladder. I changed into the gown and put my clothes in a drawstring hospital bag.

I was naked now—the bare me—in my hospital gown and socks. My heart was racing. I checked the wall clock: 6:45a.m. Several doctors, nurses, and residents came by to make their rounds—roughly, two nurses, one anesthesiologist, one colorectal resident, the colorectal surgeon, one OBGYN resident, and two OBGYN surgeons came to see me before the big dance. I signed several pieces of paper that affirmed my attestation to the procedures/ surgeries that were about to take place. Every person I met assured me that I would be taken care of throughout the process. Allen came back and sat with me as they prepared the operation room. I was hooked up to the IV, calm and terrified all at once.

Right before 7:30a.m., the nurse came to get me. I told Allen I loved him and that I would see him in a few hours. The nurse and OBGYN resident took me to the operation room. No one was there. I imagined the surgeons in the dressing area confirming everything was sterilized and putting their surgical masks and glasses on. The anesthesiologist comforted me with a few jokes about going to La La Land and told me they were going to begin strapping me in. They brought my arms out to the side and strapped me into place. Tubing was placed in my nostrils so I could get more oxygen during the surgery. Everything was happening so fast. I nodded my head, and within a few seconds, the anesthesiologist began to countdown and tell me that it would be all over soon. *Here goes nothing.* The bright lights above me begin to dim—then all went black.

My mind was the first to wake—my eyes were closed, my body limp. I heard several people talking and I felt bumps. I was moving. My eyes slowly opened a bit, then closed. All went black again for a few seconds. I was on an elevator. I felt another two bumps as the wheels of the hospital bed crossed the elevator threshold. I could hear everything distantly but I didn't feel like I was there. I heard Allen and another familiar voice, my mother-in-law, talking. I opened my eyes to say hello and raised my hand to grab theirs. Things faded out again.

I could hear but couldn't move or open my eyes. It sounded like I was in a recovery room for post-op patients. *I made it... I didn't die... Okay, that's good news*, I thought. There were Caribbean nurses/aides chatting away with their thick vibrant accents. One asked me some questions. I slitted my eyes open briefly to see her, but no words came. She walked away. I could hear the ladies complaining about their boss and chatting about what to eat for lunch. I began to slowly come to and realized, *I'm in pain. A lot of pain.* Finally, another nurse came over and I was able to open my eyes long enough to respond with head nods to her questions. She told me she would be taking me to my room shortly and to hold tight for a few minutes.

A guy came to help her and I was wheeled off to my hospital room. I fell asleep again and I woke feeling like I had been hit by 10 buses. I couldn't keep my eyes open, but managed to whisper to Allen that I needed pain meds. I assumed I had been given them because when I woke again, I was more coherent. With eyes half open, I saw hospital blankets covering my thin, petite frame. I could see the oxygen tubes in my nose, hear beeps from monitors, and a whooshing sound coming from my legs. I was unable to move much below my chest without acute pain. I glanced up and saw a curtained partition and nurses' names on the dry erase board in front of me. There was a TV in the righthand corner and my mother-in-law sat below it. Allen was standing next to her. They were chatting. I acknowledged them with a head nod and asked how long I had been in surgery. Nearly 8 hours. My eyes grew big—how was it possible to be in surgery for double the time projected by the surgeons?

"Guess what," Allen said with a heavy face.

"What!" I exclaimed as loud as I could (it was barely above a whisper).

"My dad had a heart attack at the courthouse today while you were in surgery."

"What?? What happened?"

Allen didn't have many details yet, but information was trickling in from his sister, Rena.

What a day this is shaping up to be, I told myself.

I listened to the details although I was fading in and out of awareness. I responded and slowly began to fall asleep again. My mother-in-law woke me to say she was heading back home to Pennsylvania. It was a big deal that she had taken the bus to come into the city to check on me. I was super appreciative.

The next time I woke, Allen was by my side. Now that we were alone for a minute, I pulled the oxygen tube from my nose and asked him for information on how the surgery had truly gone. The doctors believed all was successful. It had taken them longer than expected because the tumor had been so deep in the pelvic cavity. I asked about his dad and drifted back to sleep. I woke to nurses, who needed to take blood and check my vitals. Allen was getting ready to head home. He gave me a hug and was on his way.

I was terrified. I'd never spent a significant amount of time in a real hospital. I was the young person who grew up saying things like, "Thank God for medical professionals but I hate hospitals." Now, alone, I began to get reacquainted with my body. I realized that moving my abdomen was out of the question. I felt as though I was being pulled from the left and right side of my body, in opposite directions. I was sitting on my tailbone. Moving my legs felt impossible, so I wiggled my toes instead. I felt a tube between my legs, near my vagina. I would learn later that evening, when someone came by with a large measuring cup, that this was a catheter. I had been catheterized. No one had prepared me for that! I touched my belly to get familiar with the scars currently forming beneath the gauze and tape. I counted one, two, three, four, five, six sore spots across my belly.

Another surprise: I had assumed that I would have three incisions, like the last surgery, but this time it was twice that amount, indicative of the amount of work that had been done—maybe. It was as if I had gone to sleep in one body and woken up in another. *But the endo was gone.* That was what I wanted to tell myself. That was what I needed. I might not have felt good, but the monster that had been hiding in my body was gone.

A nurse came in and I asked for more pain meds. I was struggling through the pain. She later returned and injected meds into my IV. I felt relief almost instantly. I relaxed. She explained that the doctors would be by in the morning to check on my progress and someone would remove the ovary stints. *What was an ovary stint??!! Why hadn't I been told about this?* The nurse said I should get a lot of relief once those were removed. I dozed in and out over the next several hours. I only woke long enough to greet the new nurse on duty and give blood, and extend my arm and open my mouth for vitals. The night shift nurse was not nearly as kind and empathetic as the others. After my liquid dinner, I drifted off to sleep. The next day awaited and boy would it be a tough day.

7

HOLD ON

April 27. I woke with the sun, sticky, under tough sheets that had been laundered too many times. Under normal circumstances, I would have showered, washed my face, and brushed my teeth at least 3 times by then. I looked out a dusty window to see adjacent buildings and the sun easing its way through. I heard an ambulance, fire truck sirens, and a few taxis rushing by. I was exhausted because every few hours the nurses/aides would come for vitals and to give meds. However, I was optimistic and hopeful for the first time in a long time because my stomach was now flat and I didn't feel the constant pain I had felt only a few days ago. I could hear the buzz outside my door: nurses, doctors, and staff were making their morning rounds and changing shifts. Within 30 minutes, I was surrounded by new medical staff ready to take blood samples, check vitals, and measure and empty my urine. They asked me how I was feeling. I said I was fine and I complied with their requests. I still didn't feel great moving anything below my torso. The day shift nurse told me I needed to try to walk and use the bathroom on my own since it was 24 hours post-surgery. She told me to try my best and my mind settled on this new objective: walking.

The nurse asked about my pain levels. I said I could use more meds. I have an extremely high tolerance for pain, but that amount was unimaginable. She said someone would be in later in the morning from the GYN team to remove the ovarian stints, which should alleviate a lot of pressure.

I could hardly keep up with everything because every hour felt blurry. I rested a while and then heard a knock at the door. Dr. Le walked in. She asked me how I was feeling and she checked my abdomen. She told me the surgery had gone really well but the endo had been extremely deep in the pelvic cavity. (I imagined a marine biologist diving into the deep dark waters of the sea.) She said, "Be sure to try and get up and walk around today. I'll be by tomorrow to check on you."

An hour later, a nice woman from the hospital's GYN department came in with a few tools. She introduced herself and told me she would be taking my stints out and it should only take a minute. I eased down my blankets and we lifted my hospital gown. That was my first time seeing my belly. My stomach was not nearly as big and swollen as it had been a few days ago. The fibroid removal was a noticeable improvement. I laid back. She told me to take a deep breath as she pulled the left stint out first. My eyes nearly popped out of my head! I gritted my teeth, winced, and laid back. Imagine pulling a skewer out of a piece of meat or vegetable—that's what it felt and looked like. She walked around the foot of the bed to the right side to take out the other stint. I felt it slide out of my lower belly and felt instant relief. The woman dressed the two areas where the stints were and reassured me that I should feel better, and then she zipped out of the room. Now, I had a tally of 8 incisions on my belly, which I gently pressed before drifting off to sleep again.

Later in the morning, I stared at the flowers a friend had sent me and I was determined to get up and smell them. Instead of calling the nurse for help, I wrapped all my cords and the IV around my hospital gown and slowly grabbed the hospital bed rail with my left hand. With a death grip, I slowly lifted myself up and used my other hand to push my legs around the side of the bed. I released my compression pumps. Every movement was excruciating but I managed to stand on my own, hunched over like an elderly woman. My back side was exposed. How quickly appearances begin to become irrelevant when you're in a state of helplessness. I managed to make it over to the flowers to smell them with no lag left in my ropes. I realized I couldn't go too far without unhooking the numerous cords hanging from my right side, left side, and underside. After the arduous task of walking, I laid back down and I was in and out of consciousness again. In between naps, my friendly nurse came to tell me she would be back to remove my catheter and that I should attempt to void: urinate. *Sure, I have no problems peeing.* The nurse returned and lowered the bed to raise it to a comfortable height for her to help me. I helped her lift my gown and I thought, *one step closer to freedom, if this is what's needed to get out of here.* One less cord/rope too. The nurse pulled down my underwear and quickly removed the catheter. I felt free. *That wasn't so bad.* She told me to drink as much water as I could and, starting now, I had approximately eight hours to urinate. *Well, I don't need that much time.* I nodded my head and said, "Yes. Will do." I started to sip on the water and some Jello to get my bladder going.

Allen came by to sit with me for a while. He plugged in my heating pad and lifted me up to place it behind my back. After a year of needing heat as a sleep requirement, it felt amazing to enjoy it without the endo pain. We watched a show on Netflix. I told him my first night had gone well, except I hadn't slept much. Two hours later, we were in the middle of the next episode when it hit me: my belly was hurting; I needed to pee. I slowly and methodically gathered my cords and my vital signs monitor and, with Allen's assistance, I made it to the bathroom. That was my second time getting up that day, so I was feeling pretty good after the eight-hour surgery. In the bathroom, I noticed the measuring cup connected to the toilet seat. I slipped down as slowly as possible and perched onto the seat directly under the measuring cup. I sat for a bit. Nothing came out. I found this extremely odd but, without a second thought, I washed my hands and returned to the room and the Netflix show. Four hours later, I realized the pain in my pelvic cavity was increasing—*a new type of pain.* I hadn't had a trinkle come out since the catheter had been removed. I buzzed the nurse and described the pain I was feeling. She told me it was likely due to the need to urinate.

The pain increased by the second. I had drunk *a lot* of fluids. My bladder was completely full and felt like it was going to burst. My mind began to race—*I can't pee.* I tried once more with the nurse in the bathroom with me. Nothing. Panic set in. *I can't pee.* I had woken from surgery but my bladder had not. To make matters worse, the nurse told me to try to rest because I had a few more hours to attempt to void.

Throughout the evening, I doubled over in pain. Allen and I asked if I could get re-catheterized since I was in such agony. They said *no, it's best to wait and let the bladder "wake up."* I asked Allen to leave. I didn't want anyone to see me that way. You've never felt pain and suffering until you've had a full bladder and no way to empty it. I'm pretty sure you would eventually die if you couldn't release your urine.

Not a drop of urine came out. Not one drop. After hours of suffering and wincing and trying not to scream, I used the last bit of energy I had left to cry. The tears slowly dripped down my cheek and wrapped around my neck.

It was well into the evening now and I had a new night nurse: Welan. Welan had a curt personality. It was all business; nothing personal. He told me I should attempt to void once more and if nothing happened, he would be back to re-catheterize me. I told him I couldn't go and I'd tried enough. I was intensely irritated; it had been nearly eight hours—at least five hours of it spent with a full bladder. Welan told me he would be back and not to worry, that he was an expert at this. Intuitively, I knew at that moment that I should ask for a female nurse to perform the task. Besides, I had never even looked for my own urethra, let alone had a stranger dig around to find it, and stick a plastic device into it. Welan seemed confident but I was scared to death. Within 15 minutes, he was back. Just me and him in the room. Suddenly, I was shivering. On edge, I clenched my hospital gown. Welan raised the bed and told me not to worry. He put his gloves on and tore open the kit. He told me to spread my legs in the butterfly position on the bed. I slowly did as I was told, hoping the pain meds would take away any discomfort. This was the first time I'd been awake for this, so I wasn't sure what to expect.

Welan told me what he was going to do and got started. First the betadine. That was unpleasant but not unbearable. Then he pulled the tubing from the kit and spread my labia in search for my urethra. He attempted to insert the catheter and I jumped from the pain—a "don't-ever-touch-me-there-ever-again" kind of pain. He attempted again and with nervous energy told me not to move and to try to stay calm and relaxed. He attempted to insert the catheter and I winced, tensed up, and uncontrollably let out a faint "Ah!" I was trying not to scream.

Welan was determined to get the catheter in. At that point, things took a turn for the worst. I stayed still, fearful of what would happen if I didn't, but I could no longer temper my screams. His every attempt stinged more.

I broke.

"You're hurting me! Stop!!" I cried—a cry many people don't experience, and I hope never will: helpless; hopeless.

Welan tried again. Now I was screaming uncontrollably. "You're hurting me! Please stop!"

He stopped. He abruptly and shakily stopped. He dropped the catheter, told me he would bring someone else to do it, and left so fast, he appeared to be running.

I cried and drooled. The pain was unfathomable. I tried to get my heart rate back to normal as the machine monitoring it was beeping faster than ever. I felt vulnerable; violated. My bladder was still full and now my vaginal area felt battered. *Wth just happened? Why me?* I felt like an animal beaten, abused, and left for dead. I was angry at myself for not speaking up, that I hadn't gone with my gut and asked for a female nurse. Would it have made a difference if I had asked? Would Welan have complied? Would his ego and arrogance have gotten in the way? All I knew was that the experience would scar me.

Within 20 minutes, my guardian angel walked through the door: Sidney. I slowly turned my head, my eyes puffy from crying.

"I'm here to help," she said, "What happened?"

I explained the situation to Sidney and she immediately empathized with me. "I'm going to re-catheterize you. Don't worry. I'll walk you through it every step of the way." She held my hand for a while; I was inconsolable. Shaking, with tears still rolling down my face, I listened as Sidney connected with me by asking about my surgery. She said, "I'm sure you're going to feel a lot better once things settle. Sometimes guys just aren't as effective at this procedure and women are better at their own anatomy sometimes." For some reason, I trusted Sidney. She was confident but empathic. Secure, but showed vulnerability. She held my hand and told me things would be okay. "Is it okay for me to go ahead and grab another catheter kit? I'll get a smaller size as well, just in case, since you're petite." I finally calmed down and mustered, "Okay, thank you," before the tears came again. I was completely traumatized by that dreadful experience. None of it felt real; it couldn't be real.

Sidney returned, smiled, and apologized once more for what had happened. She said she was going to take care of me and peek in on me throughout my hospital stay. "Is it okay for me to get the catheter going?" she asked. I nodded through my tear-blurred vision. She lifted my gown and started to ask me questions about my life and what I do for work. I muttered a few things. Intermittently, she told me exactly what was happening down below. She applied the betadine and told me to breath out. In a split second, the catheter was inserted and the urine began to flow out. I winced from the pressure as my bladder had been stretched beyond full capacity. I began to feel relieved (literally) every second. I filled up the bin. Sidney and I both look relieved. She stayed with me for a little while longer, making small talk and making sure I was alright. "Let me know if you need anything else and I'll come by," she said.

I didn't see the night nurse anymore that evening. Whether Welan was too embarrassed to come by, I'll never know. I never wanted to see his face again.

After Sidney left, the weight of it all started to sink in. I sank further into the thin mattress and began to cry. I had woken up not expecting my bladder function to be impacted by the surgery, only to learn that it didn't work at all. That was terrifying. The remainder of the night and well into the morning, I cried. I cried because I had not been prepared for that possible post-op complication. I had the catheter experience playing repeatedly in my head. I hoped I could knock the memory out of it. I cradled my face in hopes that I could erase that nightmare. My dreams of being pain-free post-surgery had decimated. All I knew was, at this moment, I had a tube between my legs helping me to stay alive by keeping my kidneys functioning normally. I began to pray. Hard. I asked God, *why? Why did I wake up at all if this was the result?* I sobbed and sobbed.

I pulled out my air pods that were tucked beneath my pillow and began to play my tried-and-true Christian playlist. I needed hope. I didn't have ANY left. God led me to a specific song to play on my phone. I listened to it once and wept. I wanted to give in to the negative thoughts that swarmed around me like hawks. I wanted to die, but I couldn't let myself give up. All I needed was one drop of hope. With that song, I regained a tiny portion of it. I set the

song, *Hold On* (by James Fortune, featuring Monica and Fred Hammond) to
replay, over and again, until around 4a.m., when I finally drifted off to sleep.

God doesn't usually speak to us directly. Usually, He moves and speaks to
us indirectly through people. That night, He spoke to me through the words
of that song. Every single word was designed to pull me out of the depths of
despair and anguish. I could have grown bitter after the day I had had but,
instead, I held on to the words and kept my hope alive, which ultimately kept
me alive.

April 28. Many times in my life, I've noticed that sometimes you just need
to get through the night. I made it through the night and woke with hope on
my mind. *This too shall pass*, I told myself, *feelings are fleeting.* I would figure
out a way to make it. I always had. One lesson I've learned in my short years is
that you cannot depend on anyone else to encourage you. You must be your
own cheerleader. I woke up feeling relieved that the night was over and I was
hopeful for a new day. The goal for that day was to gather information on this
new condition so I could fight fair, and I was determined to get up and walk
around. I assessed my bodily condition. My eyes were puffy from the excessive
crying the night before. I gently pressed each dressing on my belly. Everything
was still in place. I touched my undies and my vaginal area, which felt very
swollen from the catheter incident, but I pushed it to the back of my mind.
I heard the usual morning buzz and I could tell the door was ajar because I
could hear more clearly.

Between 6 and 8a.m., I got the usual visits. Nurse assistants came by to
check my vitals. Sidney came by before her shift ended to check on me. I

thanked her again and told her, "You're a life saver." I really wasn't sure how I could have survived the night otherwise. My pride had been trampled. I felt stripped of dignity and my body felt like crap after that ordeal. The new nurse came by and told me she would be in at 8a.m. Everyone who popped in told me they had heard about the troubles I had had yesterday and that they were sorry it had happened... My wish came true... I never saw Welan again.

Around 8a.m., the new nurse came in and did her assessment of me. I asked her to take a look down below because everything felt swollen. She checked and her eyes widened. I explained that that was the result of last night's foolishness. I could tell she was trying not to get involved. She told me she would get ice for the swelling and it should go down in time, but to let her know if there were any changes. So, I had been right, I *was* swollen. Upset again, I was sure this was a result of the night nurse attempting to force in a catheter and pressing on sensitive nerves.

The nurse buzzed out of the room and into the room to the right of mine. In the hospital wing, I had the second-to-last room along the hall. The nurse left my door open and I could hear her conversation in the next room. I heard the unknown woman, my neighbor, ask her: "Is everything alright on the floor? Last night I heard a woman screaming and crying next door saying someone was hurting her; it was chilling, so I just wanted to make sure everything was okay." I heard the nurse respond, doing her best to reassure the patient.

So I wasn't crazy. I had been screaming and crying at the top of my lungs. Welan had assaulted me. I didn't know what to make of it. Even now, the incident is a far but clear memory. I still get chills. I recently heard the James

Fortune song again and began crying, thinking about how it had pulled me from the dark hole I had been destined for after the Day 2 post-op experiences. Should I have reported Welan? Should I have sued? I don't know. That day, all I knew was that I wanted to get better.

By mid-morning, my labia felt the size of small nectarines. I had to set that issue aside at the moment and prepare questions for my surgeon. Like clockwork, my surgeon walked in on her day off dressed in running gear. She asked me how I was feeling. I told her I was hanging on, but things hadn't been so great last night. She replied that she had heard about the catheter situation and that I was unable to void. "Have you tried again today?"

"No, not yet. I'm afraid that if I try again with the same result, someone will need to re-insert the catheter."

"That happens in some surgical cases. The tumor was so, so, so deep. It's hard to say, but the nerves in that area could have been impacted. Your bladder function will come back. Just be patient with yourself. Try again, though, today." She checked my belly, pressing around and checking the sutures. All looked good. The surgeon then patted my bed and told me she would try to check in again before I was discharged, but one of the residents would be by to check in as well. She left and I felt a bit better. *It will come back.* Now the question was *when.* My nurse buzzed in about an hour later and told me she would take the catheter out later that day so I could try again. I asked for an ice pack for my vaginal area and she brought one by. She also told me I was getting a neighbor in my room that day and to call if I needed anything, then she buzzed away.

I got up after she left, clinging to the bedrails. I wanted to walk around the halls before my new neighbor arrived. I slowly gathered my cords and pulled off my compression socks. I already felt a bit stronger. I stood on my feet and inched my way toward the door, passing the empty 2nd half of the room on my way out. *At least I have the bed by the window*, I thought. I slowly inched my way around the halls. It felt good to walk around and see what was happening outside my room. I made it to the nurses' station and one nurse came over and asked how I was doing, and if I needed help.

"No, I think I have it," I said, "but thank you."

"Take it easy and be careful." She spotted the tube of urine and she offered to grab a safety pin so I could attach the urine bag to my hospital gown. She also got an extra gown and wrapped it around me so my back wouldn't be out. I had already found a way to cover my bottom, but my back and tubes were exposed. She pinned the bag to my gown. I felt much lighter. I thanked her. "Good luck," she said, "Holler if you need anything." By then, I truly believed that everyone on the floor knew what had happened.

I kept walking. I walked around my wing and I walked around other wings of the hospital.

After 15 minutes, my body started telling me to sit down. My sutures were waking up. I turned back but felt more optimistic and encouraged.

I reached my room. There was a lot of buzz. My neighbor had arrived. She was a woman with dark hair and Eastern European features. She looked to be about 60 years old. The staff was getting her half of the room set up. I could hear her moaning and grumbling the entire time. She had just gotten out of heart surgery. I'm not certain what kind. We never spoke. I used a bit of energy to lift my hand for a slight wave but did not talk—that was forbidden; that's the New York way. I slowly and carefully got back into bed and reconnected my compression leggings. I saw I had a missed call from Allen. He was about to jump on the train and come to the hospital.

I heard the woman on her phone with a friend or her son. She grunted and groaned continuously and sounded like she'd done some smoking in her day. A courier came in and dropped off flowers from my mom. I admired the flowers and drifted off to sleep. When I woke, Allen was sitting beside me, watching TV and reading. I told him about the night I had had and how stressful it had been. I told him the full story. At this point, my vaginal area was about 3x the normal size with the swelling. Allen stood and leaned over to kiss me on the forehead and asked what he could do to help. I told him it would be nice if I could freshen up. The aids come by to refresh your linens and help you clean yourself, but it's a bit embarrassing. Allen helped by handing me the pink hospital bowl with toiletries. I began to wipe my face and brush my teeth. I looked in the mirror. I looked greasy. *Ugh. Soon I'll be out of here. I have to get out of here.*

The nurse returned and asked, "Are you ready to try to void again today? Maybe you'll have better luck this time." It was early afternoon again. She removed the catheter. I held my breath and said a prayer. I drank some water but I was cautious.

After watching a show and drifting off, I woke to find it was dark out. Allen was leaving to go and see his dad at the hospital downtown. What a week this had been. After he left, I made my way to the bathroom, easing by my neighbor. She was only interested in watching TV and defying the staff.

I sat. Still nothing. *Nothing.* I took a deep breath and pulled myself together. I couldn't keep crying. I just had to find a way to fix this. I slowly left the bathroom and realized I might as well go for a walk around the halls. The nurses kept telling me that the more I walked, the better, so that's precisely what I would do before heading back.

Our room was dimly lit with TV light and the darkness was our anguish. I sneaked over and placed a rose on my neighbor's cart while she was sleeping. No one had come to visit her. Her friend or son seemed disinterested and, based on my eavesdropping on the other side of the curtain, it sounded like she had a plethora of related health issues. I wasn't sure what my hope was with the rose, but I felt she could use cheering up. My mom always says that it's far better to give than to receive. After some pain meds, I drifted back into a solid slumber, except for the previous night's events invading my mind. I couldn't free myself from the scene that had taken place last night. I grabbed my earbuds and turned on the James Fortune song again. I let it play and I dozed off to sleep.

I was staring out of the window, watching the sun go from beaming into the room to setting on the horizon. The TV was on, but I didn't know what was on it. I was in a daze, caught between life and death, caught between loathing life and wanting to live. I thought, *why me*, more and more. I wondered if the surgery had truly been the cure I had thought it would be. Would life be better or worse now? Saddened by my extreme thoughts, I dozed off and hoped my body would fight for me because my light was dimming with every passing hour.

I woke to a jolly voice in the hallway. A woman spoke to the nurse and happily popped in, greeting me with a warm smile. She said she was a holistic wellness nurse, and she had had several surgeries and wanted to speak with me about the importance of meditation, positive thoughts, and breathing. She said we were going to meditate, that I could see myself healed. "You might not be able to see it right now," she said, "but in time, you will."

We meditated.

The wellness nurse said, "Imagine yourself at the beach, lying in the sand, and relaxing your mind and body. *Breathe.* Breathing is critical to getting better." I attempted the deep breathing techniques but felt like I was being punched in the sternum. My body felt tense and fragile, even with the pain meds. *It's in my mind*, I told myself. The nurse told me to place a pillow over my stomach and practice. The pillow helped, and I began to flow with her. Before I knew it, her time was up. She encouraged me more, then asked, "Can I come back and see you tomorrow?"

"Yes, please do. I would love that."

I tried to hold back my tears as she left the room. Optimism and hope can feel like air in a room without any. The more I received, the more I thought I could breathe. I received more hospital staff visitors and was more optimistic about the days ahead. *I have to be*, I thought to myself.

April 29. I had made it to Day 4 of post-op. That was supposed to be my last day in the hospital; however, I hadn't gone to the bathroom since I'd been there, and the staff didn't want to release me until I could go.

The morning was looking up. I got a visit from the GYN staff, Sidney, the Colorectal Chief Resident, the colorectal surgeon, and others, who were curious about my case and prognosis. I told them that despite the bladder issue, I would be okay. They told me it was significant that I'd been able to get up and move around already. Dr. Ari stopped by; he was pleased with my progress. He had come by yesterday morning (Day 3), when I could barely speak. He continued to reiterate just how deep they had had to go, but this time he explained that, because of that fact, sometimes the bladder's nerves could be adversely impacted. The nurse came in and told me there was some medicine she could give me to help me attempt to urinate. I agreed to take it because I had no choice. I didn't want to be hooked up to the catheter. Anything was better than nothing. I took the medicine and began to chug water. After an hour, I went to the bathroom. I sat and prayed that something would happen. I was sweating. Tiny beads gathered on my thin frame. I shed a tear and walked the 20 steps back to my bed. Every step hurt my body in ways I never thought I could hurt. *I am stronger than this*, I told myself. *Everything will be fine.*

Every few hours, a nurse came in to release the urine from the catheter bag into a container. Defeat chipped at my soul a bit each time.

The doctor came to tell me that I should be able to go home that day, and worst-case scenario, they would send me home with an indwelling Foley if I was still unable to void. I heard him and didn't hear him at the same time. All I knew was that if I did well that day, I could finally go home, shower, and rest. I then remembered what I had had on when I had arrived at the hospital: Lululemon tights from my first marathon and my finisher marathon pullover and sneakers. I texted Allen, asking him to find some large sweatpants so I wouldn't have to leave in a hospital gown: the weather outside was in the forties and fifties.

Uncle Ray picked my mom up from the airport. She came straight to the hospital to see me. I gave her a hug and began to cry hysterically. She sat down and I gave her the updates I could get out. She's strong, so she didn't cry with me. She said to have faith: "You must stay positive." The nurse came shortly after to tell me they would remove the catheter so I could try to go again; one last try before I went home. I could now sit more comfortably. Mom left the room to give me some privacy. I was grateful I could keep a little dignity. The nurses came in and I tried to relax my body, but I was tense. Nothing about this was glamorous. I stared out the window into the sunlight. The process was quick and painless, but not fun. After what had happened to me a few short nights ago, I was still very much on edge. One nurse touched my shoulder, said good luck, and to let them know if I needed anything. The door closed behind them.

The room was empty, and so was I, but I kept my mind focused on the light and not the darkness stirring deep within me. I sat up as tall as I could and caught up with my mom when she returned. I asked about her trip, but I could see the look of concern in her eyes as she was talking. Because she's strong, I never know what she's thinking. My face was greasy. My hair hadn't been combed. I hadn't showered since the morning I'd arrived. My mom held my hand and told me everything would be alright, to stay in faith.

I tried to urinate again, but nothing. I felt defeated, frustrated, and helpless. I slowly walked to my bed with my nurse's station attached to me; I locked eyes with my mother and shook my head.

Mental wars can be harder to fight than physical ones sometimes. I broke down with tears blurring my eyes, but I was too weak to make a sound. I fell asleep. I woke to the nurse on duty coming in to share that I should be able to go home that night. They needed the doctors to sign off on some things, then we could go.

I attempted to go again, and suddenly, a few drops trickled out. *Hallelujah!* My mom was right. I had to stay positive. The nurse came in to check the bathroom and didn't see any urine, so she knew, but she had to ask... I shook my head, "Yes, a little came out!"

"Great," the nurse said, "that's good news but we have to catheterize you before you go, since it wasn't very much." I looked up and nodded.

My bladder was bursting at the seams. They brought a lady team in and got me ready. My mom stayed this time to hold my hand. She spoke encouragement into the room, and I was good to go in a few minutes. The tape was secure, and the catheter bag was taped around my thin leg. I could relax now. How quickly the human species can adjust; it's fascinating. For the first time, and very quickly, the bag brought me comfort. Only those who've experienced what it is like to not be able to relieve yourself can understand this. You will die if you can't relieve yourself. There is no way around it.

Allen came to the hospital to meet us. That morning I had asked him to go to Century 21 and buy men's sweatpants for me, so they could cover the catheter. This wasn't how I had envisioned my trip home, but things don't always work out the way we plan them.

We waited. About an hour later, the nurse said, "Good news, you can pack up and get ready for discharge. I will need to remove your IVs and monitors." As the nurses started to remove the equipment, I felt one step closer to freedom. "Call me when you are ready to go," the nurse said. I'd been there for four days and I could barely rev my engine to stand, but I did it somehow—one foot in front of the other. I stood and started bossing everyone around, rushing them to hurry and pack me up. I laughed at the looks I received from my mom and Allen as I directed them on how to pack for me. I couldn't wait to get home and lay in my own bed.

I removed the hospital gown, peered down at myself, and shrugged it off. There were stitches everywhere, it seemed, but I didn't care. I could finally go home. The worst was over. Allen and Mom's eyebrows furrowed at me. "You're moving too fast in your condition," they said. In my head, I was moving too slowly. I finally called the nurse's line and said, "I'm ready for discharge." The seconds seemed like minutes, and minutes like hours. Finally, a Caribbean nurse told me she was there to review my discharge instructions. She sat on the bed beside me and reviewed each page in detail. *Make sure you do...* I agreed and signed. At 9:25p.m., after four days of internal healing, pain, frustration, anger, sadness, weeping, and struggle, I was officially discharged from Lenox Hill Hospital.

I was free! I was closer to recovery and real rest. The nurse told me my wheelchair would be up momentarily. I sat and waited. For the first time, I felt calm. My chariot arrived and I was wheeled down the hall I'd painfully walked over the past few days. I nodded at the nurses as I went by. I had a much stronger appreciation for hospital staff than ever before. Some names and faces will remain with me forever.

My wheelchair driver told my family we would meet them on the ground floor level. He wheeled me into an elevator and each bump felt like a knife to the stomach. We quickly arrived at the front door, and before I knew it, I was outside in the spring NYC air. It was cold and windy. I was eased into the back of an SUV, and we were off. The hospital lights went by in a blur, then they were behind me. I was on my way home. For the first time, I was also relieved for my family. This was taxing on them, and I felt blessed to have them. Every bump in the Uber ride felt like a punch, but I curled up, braced my arms around my midsection, and tried to enjoy the view. The city lights glistened off the water as we hugged the FDR toward the Brooklyn Bridge. Freedom never felt so good. We arrived home around 10p.m., and I immediately asked for help getting into the shower. My mom helped me, and I stood under the water for a minute. Every movement felt as though I was relearning it for the first time, but I took my time and gritted through. I stepped out of the tub, smiling from ear to ear. Mommy nurse helped me into bed, and I smiled. I was home.

8

RECOVERY ROAD

April 30. My eyes opened to the beautiful bright sun gleaming through my window from our high-rise apartment. I could move my head with ease, but the rest of my body needed to be retrained. I slowly shifted around to stare out the window. Tears wanted to well up, but I took a deep breath. I could genuinely smile for the first time in nearly a week. I looked at my nightstand and grabbed the orange pill bottles to see what was on the agenda for today. I'm strong, but I knew I needed to follow the discharge instructions and take Tylenol and Oxy immediately to get ahead of the pain. I felt dull stabs across my abdomen. My belly felt hollow and stiff, like it needed a lot of time to wake up. I knew recovery would take a while.

I had my water cup from the hospital. I grabbed it and gulped down my new regimen: Tylenol; Oxy; Colace. In the next room, I heard pots and pans clanking and the smell of Mom's breakfast. I smiled big, then slowly and painstakingly glided my legs toward the edge of the bed. I got both feet planted on the floor, one leg at a time, and I lifted my gown to check out my new accessories.

My urine bag was a gut punch, a downer, but I reminded myself that this was a fight and I was not backing down. The bag was there, but not there to stay. I checked my incisions and most looked okay. One looked gross, but I could do nothing but take it easy and let things heal. With one hand railing the bed, I opened the door. My mom said, "Good morning, Sleeping Beauty. How are you feeling? Who told you to get up by yourself?!" She's always fussing at me but for a good cause. "I'm fine," I told her, in that eye-roll teenager kind of way, "I'm going to the bathroom." She stopped to help me make the 5-10-step journey. Thankfully, I had a small chair/stool in my bathroom. I emptied my bag into the toilet and flushed. I washed my hands and face and brushed my teeth. When I came back out, my mom had a full spread ready for me.

I was supposed to be on a low-fiber diet. Grits weren't disqualified, so this southern girl was happy about that! I sat and watched Good Morning America with my mom and ate. Pillows propped me up on all sides but, for the first time, things were normal. A new normal, but normal nonetheless, and that's all I could ask for. I ventured into the hallway with my mom and did a few laps around the floor. I started with one lap and tried to increase it a little each day. I had a cane in one hand and leaned on her with the other for support. Every step felt like climbing Mt. Everest, but I knew I had to do this. I didn't have a choice. There was too much life to be lived and I wanted to see it. When I felt sad or wanted to cry, my mom would interject with an encouraging word. I was learning to accept the process. It was my journey and I had to own it. This was my routine over the next couple of days: wake up; take meds; spend time assessing myself in the bathroom; eat three meals a day at least (thanks, Mom);

do breathing exercises; and rest in bed.

As I mentioned at the beginning of this book, I am highly ambitious (aka, stubborn). As I planned for surgery, I told my boss I would be back in one week, on May 6th. I'd been checking my email the entire time and checking in with my coworkers who were covering my projects, to give guidance. As the week winded down, I quickly realized one week was a ridiculous farce. I reluctantly sent an email to HR, and then, within minutes, I was on the phone with Kacy from HR. I explained everything to her and tried not to sob to a stranger. I like living in my superhero world where everything is great, everyone is strong, and nothing bad happens to good people, but when I had to share my story, it became more real. Kacy reassured me that everything would be okay and she would take care of everything. She told me I had benefits, which was why the company paid insurance: so we could use it when needed. I could expect to have 90 days for recovery at 80% of my salary. She sent me the short-term disability paperwork and told me to fill it out ASAP so she could send it to Prudential. Kacy kept her word and became another one of my guardian angels. I relaxed a bit more.

By Friday, May 3rd, I was beginning to get into a routine, but I was noticing that it hurt to sit down—it really, really hurt. I could barely sit on the couch without extreme pain to my tailbone. Thankfully, we lived in NYC. I seriously believe there isn't much you can't find there. Allen called a few local pharmacies and found a donut cushion for me on his way home from work. I sat and it was such a relief. It wasn't perfect, but I could now sit for over fifteen minutes without being in agonizing pain. I could feel my tailbone throbbing. I was already thin, but I'd lost more weight since the surgery. We ate the dinner my mom had prepared and found a movie to watch.

I constantly shifted around, but I looked at my mom and Allen. Gratitude was the only word I could think of to describe the primary feeling driving me forward. They had no idea how I was feeling mentally or physically, but they were there for me. When your physical health becomes endangered, you rethink everything and look at life through new eyes. Life is fragile. Relationships are a treasure. Laughter is a gift. Material things become meaningless. You begin to live, not looking with your eyes through your body, but looking with your soul through your spirit. I laughed and enjoyed the movie. *I am going to be okay*, I told myself. For the first time, I really meant it.

On Saturday, I woke up feeling invigorated. I decided to cut out the Oxy because my pain was manageable now with just Tylenol. So, I was down to Tylenol and Colase. The surgeons' offices had called a few times to check in.

I decided on sweats and a sweatshirt that day. I would not be wearing leggings or jeans in the foreseeable future. I could do most of the basics on my own, but walking more than 20 steps was still challenging.

We spent the day watching shows and movies and ordering takeout. I went into the hall for my usual walks and ventured into the stairwell. Progress! I went up and down a few steps and was sweating by the time I got back to the apartment. I had seriously underestimated my recovery! The three months of short-term disability seemed more reasonable every day. At this point, I was down to one nap per day. Things were looking up.

9

"NO LUCK"

On Sunday, May 5th, I spent time with my family and enjoyed sitting on the donut in my work chair because the couch still wasn't an option. My abdomen was very fragile. We ordered Mexican food in the evening, played games, and watched movies. By the end of the night, in typical project manager form, I checked my schedule for the week. I needed to see a urologist, GYN surgeons, and my colorectal surgeon. I was looking forward to getting out of the apartment and getting back into the streets to feed off the city energy.

First up was the urologist appointment. I lived in Downtown Brooklyn, and the office was on Manhattan's Upper East Side. Based on my attempt at taking the stairs during my daily walks, I quickly eliminated the subway as a means of transportation. I charted out when we needed to leave and I went to sleep early. Tomorrow would be a big day and I needed to be ready. I said my prayers and stared out into the twinkling city lights or, as I like to call them, NYC stars. The twinkles began to grow dull as I fell fast asleep.

On Monday, May 6th, I woke up and eagerly got dressed. My mom and

I looked at each other and headed out the door. I had no clue what to expect as I'd never been to a urologist before. Hell, before this year, I hadn't been to many doctors at all. We got in the elevator and pushed the button for the lobby. People piled into the elevator on the way down with their dogs, gym clothes or laptop bags, going about their normal lives. We reached the lobby, and I was the last one out with my mom. The building staff all had looks of surprise and relief. They were used to me waving with a huge smile every morning and rushing out like my legs were catching fire. Now, my neighbors had already zipped out, and the doors were closed behind them before I even got close. Tom, the doorman, nodded respectfully and put his head down. I gave a slight wave and half grin, and the doors opened to the NYC sun and wind.

The cars and taxis whirled about, and pedestrians were buzzing. The hum of the streets made me feel tired. Our Uber arrived and my mom held my arm tightly and helped me to the car. It was 11 days since surgery, but felt like yesterday. The car door opened and I was suddenly stuck figuring out how to ease inside without worsening the pain. I couldn't lift my leg, so I sat first instead. That was better. My mom helped me lift one leg at a time until I was in. I had the bag between my legs, so I slowly adjusted to avoid a leak. My mom walked around, and within seconds we were off. I smiled at the driver out of decency and held on to whatever my hands could find to brace. My mom patted my hand, and we squeezed each other's hand before letting go. I stared out the window as we buzzed towards DUMBO and over the Brooklyn Bridge to the FDR. It was still one of the most beautiful views I'd ever seen.

We made our way into the Upper East Side, where there is always some

great people-watching from a cab. Older women with their pups strolled lei-
surely. Huge trucks unloaded inventory for restaurants. Business people on
their phones grabbed coffee from the local baristas. Young people had their
headphones on, in their cocoons. Older people walked the streets getting their
exercise. Nannies walked strollers to Central Park before and during naptimes.
We pulled up to the office and I slowly got out of the car. The Uber flew off in
a hurry and we were left on a quiet street full of offices.

I walked in and gave the receptionist my name and info. She told me to
have a seat and that she would be right with me. She fussed on the phone with
someone's insurance provider then called me back up. I filled out the neces-
sary information and she told me that the doctor would be with me shortly.
My mother and I sat and watched the TV. They were playing the Netflix show
with Jerry Seinfeld driving around NYC with comedians.

After twenty minutes or so, I was called into the office. The urologist's
office was filled with photos and articles and it was very messy, not what I
was accustomed to seeing, but whatever. He asked me to give him the details
again. I relived the events of the last week and a half. He said, "It will come
back. Your bladder needs to wake up, and it takes time. It will come back.
Today, let's take the catheter out and give you a couple of hours to try to go.
Come back to my office if you can't. Here, here's my cell. Call me later. Let me
know how it's going." He pointed to the door of the exam room and asked me
to go in and have a seat; he would be in shortly with his assistant.

I went to the room and sat on the examination table. After a few minutes, the doctor and his assistant (a woman in her late twenties) came in. He
got a pair of gloves and told me, "This won't hurt at all. You may feel a bit

of pressure." I laid completely flat on the table and squeezed my hands together. Within seconds, the catheter was removed. He popped the gloves off and told me to call him later, and hurried out of the door, back into his office. The assistant came behind him to remove the medical-grade tape from my thigh. She apologized for the discomfort. Within a minute, the tape was also gone. She tossed the catheter and all associated accessories into the trash bin. I was feeling so much relief and so much lighter without the bag. The assistant grabbed my arms and helped me to sit up. "You're free to go," she said. "Let us know how it goes. Good luck."

I walked back into the waiting room and signaled to my mom that we could go. She immediately asked, "So what happened? What did he say?" I told her he wanted me to try to go again and to come back if I needed to, but otherwise, we could go home if I was able to void. She said, "Okay, well, let's roll." I was eager to try now.

We walked toward Central Park and I found someone selling water. I bought two bottles and we continued strolling and chatting about the things we saw along the way. Some city wildlife (squirrels and birds). Little kids running around and dogs galore. Runners getting in midday runs around the park. I finished one bottle of water and we found a bench to rest. We chatted for the next thirty minutes. It felt great leaving the apartment and walking around with less baggage. My mom and I were secretly praying hard for a win that day. After about an hour, we got up and walked a bit more, and she asked the question I'd been thinking the entire time but hadn't wanted to answer in reality: "Do you feel like you have to go?"

I shook my head. "Not yet."

"Okay, let's keep walking, if you can."

We walked North. I showed her where my GYN's office was, as it was only a few blocks north of the urologist. In silence, I stopped and bought another bottle of water along the way. I take some sips because I didn't want to fill up too quickly. I didn't feel a thing yet, and we were quickly approaching two hours. As we walked on, we came upon a much-needed distraction. There were barricades and people were sitting on the streets. We got closer and realized we were across the street from the Metropolitan Museum of Art. Today was the Met Gala! Earlier in the park, I'd thought I'd seen a woman pushing Serena Williams' daughter in a stroller, but figured there was no way that was her daughter. Maybe it had been!

We leaned against a building and watched for a while. The entrance area was gorgeous. People with passes/badges were zipping in, out, and around, setting up. Young people were camped out with pillows and snacks and taking turns going to the restroom. Though this distraction was needed, it didn't take away the thoughts in the back of my mind. I didn't feel *anything*. We walked toward Lexington Avenue and made our way to the Nespresso shop. I tried to go, but nothing, so we left; I was too tired to go on now. I dug into my crossbody and took out the business card with the doctor's cell number handwritten on the back. I dialed the number and he answered within a few rings.

"Hi, this is Crystal. I was in your office a few hours ago. I've had fluids and tried, but no luck voiding."

"Are you sure you don't want to give it more time?"

"No. I'm sure I don't feel anything, but I can tell my bladder is full."

"Come back in when you're ready," he said.

I felt defeated, but luckily we had a cool distraction around. My mom and I were on a block with black SUVs and paparazzi near a boutique hotel. Some claimed Kim Kardashian was upstairs getting dressed for the Met Gala. We discussed the pomp and circumstance on our way back to the office. When we arrived on the street, it was an entirely different environment. No energy and somewhat lifeless which, unfortunately, was precisely how I felt, though I was trying to control my emotions. I knew I would be going home with another catheter and urine bag.

Inside the office, the assistant came to get me. She told me they would clear the urine first and reinsert the catheter, that I would be in and out in no time. I braced for the experience and mainly focused on the assistant. She was warm and helpful, as if she 100% empathized with the situation. I slowly felt the pressure in my belly going down. It's a strange sensation to not have the ability to feel yourself going. But feeling pressure being released let me know how uncomfortable I had actually been over the last few hours. The doctor told me he was all done and "Let's try again in a few days. Come back on Friday." I told him I would, and his assistant helped me up again. I sincerely thanked her as she taped the bag back to my leg. Everything wasn't secure this time because I'd had the hospital-grade tape for the last seven days. The bag moved every step I took. I headed out to the waiting room to my mom.

"I'll be back in a few days," I said.

"Well, we believe everything will be better by then."

"Please God. I hope so."

We made our way out into the sun and waited for the Uber to arrive. There was so much relief knowing I was going home. I did what I always did: I stared out the window at the sea of people, cars, and tall buildings, distracting myself from reality, if only for a moment.

After 5 hours walking the streets of the Upper East Side of Manhattan, I was back home in my Brooklyn apartment, relieved there was a way to relieve myself and death was off the table again. I stared out the window as my mom whipped us up a dinner plate. I ate and smiled as if I was okay, and I was, somewhat. I was so exhausted from the walking that I eased into bed after dinner, tuned the TV to the Met Gala, and watched the stars walk the carpet and show the world their chosen looks. My mom and I discussed the various looks through the door as she watched from the other room. I couldn't be more grateful for the distraction. Eventually, I turned my head away and fell asleep to the debates about the best couture.

The next day I woke up to my usual rituals and felt invigorated. Today was post follow-up with the gynecological surgeons. I felt a bit more prepared and ready. Fewer nerves. I smiled a little brighter at the front desk attendant in the building lobby and attempted to walk a little taller. We hopped in an Uber and headed uptown again. I stared out my window at Brooklyn as we raced up the FDR. Everything still hurt, but now I was learning how to manage. We arrived and walked in the short hallway to the office door. We went in, and I suddenly felt at ease, as if I was safe and understood. Everyone there was rallying around the same cause. One purpose: getting help with endo or helping someone with endo. I signed in and my mom grabbed a magazine and flipped through it. I remembered that there had been someone post op the last time I had been there, and she could barely get around. I got it now. I don't know what stage of the disease she had, and it didn't matter. It crushes you and your spirit in a way only a select few can understand.

I was eventually called and placed in a room so the doctors could see how I was healing.

"How are you, Crystal?" asked Dr. Le. "You've been through a lot. How are you recovering? Any changes?" She checked the incisions and applied some pressure to my abdomen. "Everything looks good. Do you still have the Foley?"

"I saw Dr. Roberts yesterday."

"Oh good. How did it go?"

"He removed the Foley, and I walked around for a few hours with my mom, but no luck. I couldn't feel anything."

"Okay. Ugh, I know that is frustrating for you. This happens in a small percentage of surgeries performed... The endo was so extensive that we had to go so deep ... sometimes the nerves are impacted. Don't worry; it will come back. These things can take time. When do you go back to see him?"

"I go back on Friday."

"Okay, good."

She asked me other questions about the pain level I was experiencing, and explained that the other surgeon had to prepare for the big conference they host each year, so he couldn't make it to the appointment. I told her that's understandable, and that I appreciated her support throughout this process and for doing such a wonderful job. We chatted about her running. Oh, how I wished I could run away from all this, but I was living this out one day at a time. After a sigh of relief, and comfort from talking with the surgeon, I returned to the waiting area, waved at my mom, and said my goodbyes to the ladies at the front desk. They'd been such a tremendous help. Inside me, tears began to form. I took one more look at the office and closed the door behind me, hoping I never needed to return. Outside, I told my mom about my conversation with the doctor, and we slowly pivoted to talking about something else. We enjoyed the air and walked until I couldn't walk anymore, then we hailed a taxi to take us home.

May 8, 2019.

A better day. Mom made a light breakfast for me, and we watched TV. Sitting still hurt, but I was learning to cope with the pain. I wasn't sitting on the couch because I still needed abdominal support. We watched the news and GMA and went into the hallway for a morning turn about the hall. I motioned to my mother that I could go on my own now—without leaning on her as a crutch. I was getting better and better. Every step gave me hope. I told my mom, "Hey, let's get some fresh air." I wanted to take the stairs to the rooftop. It was only a few flights of stairs, but it might as well have been 20 flights for me at the time. Each step was painful, but it was worth the try. By the time we made it up, I was winded, but when the air hit my face and the sun touched my eyes, I quickly forgot about it. We were the only ones there because it was the middle of the day on a Wednesday. We looked out into the distance at the Staten Island bridge, and I got flashbacks of running across it in the NYC Marathon, and how it had felt breaking through the wind, letting it carry me, pushing me forward. I felt inspired and decided to sit with that memory for a bit. Sometimes we need our past successes to give our future hope.

We eventually headed back down to the apartment, but on the elevator this time. After an evening of laughter, everyone prepared for bed. I stayed up a while and thought about the future. I was ready to get back to my old life. I told myself to be patient. I said my prayers, popped in my AirPods, and listened to the audiobook by TD Jakes called *Crushing*. I eventually nodded off to sleep.

May 9, 2019.

This was supposed to be my last doctor's visit for the week. I needed to follow up with Dr. Ari, the colorectal surgeon. This time, my riding partner and I were heading to Midtown. We get out of the Uber and were immediately encapsulated by the pulsing energy of Midtown Manhattan. Everyone walks fast and bagel stands are on every corner. I had worked only a few blocks from there a few years ago. I was surrounded by my peers texting with one hand and holding salads in the other hand. We cut through the sidewalk traffic to get to the building entrance. We headed up to the 6th floor, and all was quiet. I sighed deeply, signed in, and sat. The TV was on one of those afternoon judge shows. I watched a bit and thought about topics I wanted to share. I hadn't told my family, but I'd been having some embarrassing issues since the surgery that I had been too sad and ashamed to talk about.

"Ms. Brown!" the nurse yelled, as if the waiting area is an auditorium. I love New Yorkers. Loud and assertive. She smiled, and I eased up from the chair with both hands planted firmly on the armrests. The nurse took me back to the one exam room the doctor had. She checked my vitals and told me the doctor would be right in. Within a minute, the doctor came in and said: "It's good to see you. How are things going?"

"Overall, okay. Much better. But I can feel the area where the surgery was performed because I can feel the ring when I go to the bathroom. I still have the Foley right now. And I see a small amout of stool in my underwear when I go to the bathroom." I'd admitted it. I held back the tears I'd been fighting for the past several days. I sucked them back in so the doctor wouldn't see them. He told me he needed to check where he'd fused the rectum back together. I winced at the thought of it, considering I was still not well enough to use my abs, let alone let someone check out an area where I could feel internal soreness. He left the room and told me to lie on the table, and that he would be back in a few.

I lay on the bed facedown and tried not to move. I heard a knock on the door. Dr. Ari and his female assistant were back in the room. The assistant helped me roll my sweatpants down, and I heard the sound of gloves being pulled from a box.

The doctor said, "I'm just going to check the site. I know this is unpleasant after surgery, but I have to make sure everything is healing well... You will feel a warm gel. Try to relax." He checked things out, and I gritted my teeth. He felt the circle and snapped the gloves off and into the trash. "Everything appears to be healing well." The assistant helped me sit and pull my pants back up. The doctor continued, "I don't feel anything abnormal, so our best bet is to take it easy and rest as much as possible so things can begin to heal. Regarding the other matter, things should improve with time, but your surgery was very extensive, so you'll have to be patient. Take a fiber supplement if you need to and continue to take your Colace in the meantime. I want to see you back in a month or so. Call my office if you need anything or if your symptoms worsen. When do you see Dr. Roberts again?"

"Tomorrow."

"Okay, good. It will come back, but it could take some time for your bladder to wake up."

Again, I held back tears and nodded my head to signal an agreement.

I walked slowly down the hall to the checkout desk. The ladies were scurrying around: one answering calls; one checking people in; and one checking people out. The nurse handed my file to the checkout clerk and said, "Okay, Ms. Brown, let's get you on the calendar for your next appointment." We set a date and exchanged pleasantries.

Before opening the waiting room door, I replaced my downtrodden face with a brave one. I smiled and said to my mom, "Let's roll." She got up and asked (of course): "How did it go?" I told her it went well. We walked out, and I was happy to be outside and distracted so I could tuck away the tears threatening to fall. I had to be brave, strong, and have faith. I had to do everything I could to get well. That was my only goal. We walked around Midtown and fed off the energy before hailing a cab back to Brooklyn.

My mom was flying out the next day. I was emotional about it. I was so grateful that she had come to stay with me that week. I needed her support, her laughter, and her joyful energy. I held back tears. I was a bucket of tears those days and it was super frustrating. But how can you go through a surgery that extensive and not get emotional? I was alive, in pain, but not endometriosis pain. I could now sleep without painkillers and opioids—a new feeling. I thought about all the women who had endo and didn't know it, and it sickened me and created a sense of pure hopelessness. *I have to do something one day*, I told myself. Mom and I sat around and watched some of her favorite shows until I couldn't sit anymore.

Three appointments down, and one more to go that week. I was so nervous about the next day, I could hardly breathe. I prayed hard, hoping that would somehow speed things up and my bladder would work better than ever the next day. I lay in bed and envisioned my bladder working. I imagined a future where I was better and happy.

I believe God hears every prayer, feels our every emotion, and sees every tear. We might not audibly hear from him, but there are signs we ignore and take for granted. Your eyes open the next day. You see a beautiful sunset. Birds chirping. Smiling people. The laughter of children at play. *All things work together*, I told myself. *Why am I so emotional?* I processed my emotions and realized I'd never been so out of control before. But I had no control whatsoever of this situation. I was at the mercy of the Master of the Universe. I prayed as hard as I could and, per my usual routine, drifted off to sleep with tears gliding down my cheekbone to my ears.

May 10, 2019.

A big day. My mom was flying home to Georgia in the early afternoon, and I had to go back to the urologist that day—alone.

Allen woke around 6a.m. and asked, "How do you feel about today?"

"I don't know. Nervous, I guess."

"Don't be nervous. You got this. Everything is going to be okay. You're going to heal. Call me if you need me." He kissed my forehead, caressed my hair, and went into the closet to put on his banker uniform, and into the bathroom to get ready for work.

He hugged my mom and said thank you.

"Take care of her now," she said, and patted his arm.

Allen ran out the door yelling, "Call me later!" I heard the door slam and I took a deep breath.

My mom hugged me when I finally came out of the bedroom and asked in her *goo-goo-ga-ga* voice, "Are you going to be alright? Do I need to move my flight for Mama's baby?"

"No, no, no. I'll be fine," I smiled.

She was packing up. I headed to the bathroom to empty my Foley bag. My new morning routine included emptying my bag, washing my hands and face, brushing my teeth, and checking my scars/incision sites. I looked in the mirror and told myself: *I can do all things. I'm strong. I'm brave. I'm courageous. I'm healing well.* I took a deep breath and walked to my closet to get changed. I was ready.

I placed my shoulder bag over my thin frame and grabbed fruit from the kitchen. I gave my mom a big hug, thanked her again for everything, and said, "I'll let you know how things go. Keep me posted on your flight. Talk to you later. Love you." I closed the door behind me and put my earbuds in. I hit the elevator with more confidence than I'd had all week. I was on my own now.

I headed into the city and uptown once again for the last time that week. I crossed Flatbush and hopped into a budget ride-share service, only in NYC, that uses a van to pick up people along a route, like a bus. The Ubers, to and from the city that week, had been adding up fast, and I knew I was in no condition to attempt the train just yet.

After 45 minutes in the van, I texted Allen and asked him to call the urologist's office and tell them I was running 30 minutes behind. In NYC, convenience costs. A lot. Saving $15-$20 made me 40 minutes late for my appointment. I didn't let much stress me those days, I was dealing with enough. I arrived at 10:20a.m. and signed in. The same Netflix show was streaming on the TV in the waiting room. Jerry Seinfeld and a new comedian this time. I glanced up occasionally to watch, and checked my work email app to keep a pulse on what was happening. I hadn't sent a single email since going on short-term disability. I had bigger fish to fry.

"Ms. Brown, come with me," said the assistant.

Using only my legs, I eased up as straight as possible and hobbled into one of the rooms.

"The doctor and I will be in with you shortly," the assistant said.

After about 15 minutes, the doctor came in and said, "What are we doing today? Removing the Foley so you can try again, correct? ...Okay, let's do it." He popped on his gloves and the assistant helped me lie flat on the exam table. The catheter was out within a minute; I was free again. "Okay," the doctor said, "hopefully I don't see you, but if you can't go, call me and head back to the office."

He left to let the assistant remove the tape that had been glued to my leg all week.

"Okay, that's it," she said, "Let us know how it goes."

I dressed and walked out into the sunshine. I was prepared today and had brought my own water, which I sipped as I walked. I went to Central Park and observed everything and everyone. I walked down to Central Park Zoo and further down until I neared 5th and 59th. I went into a Pret nearby and grabbed a sandwich to snack on. I didn't feel anything, but it had only been a little over an hour. I had time. I found a bench and watched birds scrounge for food on the sidewalks, and between cracks and crevices near food carts.

I drank more water and began to head uptown. I had nothing but time. Eventually, I made my way back up to the Metropolitan Museum of Art, and everything was back to normal post-Met Gala. I observed the people, the doormen, and the construction workers, all busy and scurrying about. I watched wealthy older people walking their dogs and getting fresh air.

The sun was getting high, and I began to get tired. I walked slower. I had to go somewhere and try. I found a busy restaurant and tried, but not a drop. I felt my bladder weighing me down more and more with every step, and I started to hold my belly. I called Allen. He'd rented a car and would pick me up and take me home that day. He was leaving the office early. It was the Friday before Mother's Day weekend, so he had planned to visit his mom the next day.

I made my way back down to the urologist's office, arriving around 2p.m. I told the assistant, "No luck." She gave me a look that was enough to warrant a verbal thank you. "I'll let Dr. Roberts know."

I sat and waited. My bladder hadn't wakened. *Will it ever? Will I always need this bag on my leg?* I dragged my mind away from the rabbit hole.

I saw the doctor again. "No luck, huh? ...It will come back. It always does. These things take time. Come back and see me in a week or two."

They released the urine, funneled it into a jug, replaced the catheter and the dreaded bag, and taped the bag to me again. When they left the room, I stared at my left leg—skinny and frail with tape securing a piece of my lifeline. I didn't cry. I got up and left.

The sun was still bright in the sky. Around 4p.m., Allen picked me up, and I eased into the car, relieved to be going home. *What a week*, I thought, *but at least it's over.* I was faring well overall, and that was still something.

I enjoyed the sun and the breeze as we crossed the Brooklyn Bridge. That was my new normal, and that was okay. I might not have liked it, but I had to keep moving. *If sharks don't swim, they die*, I told myself. *If you don't keep moving, you die.*

Back at the apartment, I showered, changed into comfortable clothes, and piled onto the couch. My mom had landed safely back home and things seemed to be looking up. The evening sky was beautiful, and I was grateful to my support system for keeping me sane and distracted.

Allen wrapped up a work call, showered, and changed into comfy clothes, too. We both piled up on the couch for the first time in weeks.

I lay on my right side to avoid tailbone pain. "Thank you for sticking with me through this, love. I know it hasn't been easy, but I think things are smoothing out from here," I said.

"It's my job. I got you."

We browsed Netflix for a movie, placed a takeout order, cracked open a window to hear the sound of Brooklyn in the background, and got a cool spring breeze. A good day.

10

DEATH'S DOOR

May 11, 2019. I woke, turned over in bed, and before I could open my eyes, a jolt of pain shot through my abdomen. My eyes popped open. I winced, sat up, and grabbed my stomach.

"What's up? Everything okay?" Allen asked.

"I don't know. My lower abdomen hurts really bad. Maybe it's bladder spasms?"

"Let's keep an eye on it."

I lay back down. The pain was so sudden and throbbed relentlessly.

Allen got up and dressed for the gym. He would be heading out of town to visit his mom. It was Mother's Day weekend. I cheered him on while I tried not to move because of the severe pain. Before Allen left, he said, "Reach out to Dr. Le and let her know what's going on."

"Okay," I said, reluctantly, "Don't worry about me." The pain was not letting up no matter if I lay, sat, or stood.

I stood up and my knees buckled. Then I was on the floor holding onto the bed with one frail hand. My hand shook as I grabbed my phone and pulled up Dr. Le's contact info and sent her a text:

Hi Dr. Le. This is Crystal Brown (surgery 2 weeks ago). Dr. Roberts replaced the Foley yesterday. I've had tough bladder spasms/sharp pains. Any recommendations? It's pretty severe.

Two minutes later she responded and asked me a few questions about my current meds. I told her which ones I'd taken since I'd left the hospital: Ketorolac 10mg and Phenazopyridine 200mg. Both were gone. I had taken them, along with an opioid and Colase, since leaving the hospital. She prescribed some bladder spasm and pain meds immediately. *This woman is a God-send*, I thought. I chuckled to myself: *If it not one thing, it's another.* I reached out for my cane, slowly rose from the floor, and walked into the bathroom.

I could barely move, but I pushed through. I sat on the stool in our bathroom and sent Allen a text:

Can you run by the pharmacy and pick up some meds Dr. Le called in please? The one in Target.

I showered, threw on a big shirt, and lay back down. A text from Allen popped in:

Hey. Pharmacy isn't open until 11.

We exchanged a few text messages and within minutes I heard the apartment door slam shut behind Allen. He said, "Just have the doctor send them to the one down Flatbush."

"No, she's done enough. I don't want to inconvenience her. I'll go get them myself at 11. I'm sorry, I should have checked."

"You'll go get them? Uhh, no you won't. You don't need to go anywhere." He slowly sat down on the bed as if I might break and looked at me for a while. I didn't like that, so I said, "What is it? What are you looking at? I feel like you're staring into my soul."

"I am. You don't look right and I'm staying here today."

"No! You need to go see your mom! It's Mother's Day weekend and she's expecting you."

"I know, and I get that, but you don't look right and I'm not leaving you here alone. I'll go and get the meds at 11. My mom will understand. I'll call her shortly and I may still go tomorrow."

I said okay, but inwardly I felt like such a burden. I tried to put it out of my mind.

At 11a.m., Allen ran to the pharmacy to pick up my prescriptions. I heard the door slam and I hopped up to meet him in the kitchen. I grabbed some water and immediately popped open the brown paper bag. Dr. Le had prescribed some bladder spasm refills and a pain med to help. I take all three as recommended and lay down on the couch. Allen and I spent the afternoon binging a show as I fell in and out of sleep. Before long, the sun was beginning to go down. When I woke and peeked out, the sky was a beautiful light orange and blue. I woke for a little bit to ask what I had missed Allen laughed and got me up to speed on the show "we were" watching. I faded back out for a bit and the next time I woke it was 6:45p.m. I immediately felt cold and pulled a blanket down from the back of the couch. I stared over at Allen thinking about how blessed I was to have him with me.

I took a photo of him and he smiled. I thanked him again for spending the day with me because I knew this hadn't been the plan for the day. He grabbed my hand and said, "Stop apologizing. It's all good." His face changed from a smile to a frown after a few seconds. "Why are your hands so cold?"

"I don't know. I'm freezing all of a sudden. Can you bring me another blanket? ...Better yet, I'm going to go and get into bed and get under the covers for a bit." I used Allen's strong arms as leverage to help me up off the couch. "I'll be fine," I said, responding to the worry in his eyes, "I just need to rest in bed." He helped me into bed and I pulled the sheet and duvet over my shoulders and put the TV on for background noise. After a few minutes sitting with my eyes closed, I realized I was shivering. I grabbed the blanket at the base of our bed and pulled it up to my shoulders.

A few minutes passed and I called out to Allen, asking him to bring the blanket from our couch for me. He walked into the room and looked at me as if he had just seen a ghost. His movements slowed as he stared and gently lay the blanket across the bed, over my thin, shaking body. "We need to check your temperature," he said.

I didn't protest.

Allen returned with a thermometer. 101.3. I looked at him. "I feel fine, don't worry so much. I'm just cold and a bit sleepy."

"I'm calling the doctor on call."

"NO! You know what they are going to say. They will want me to go to the hospital. I can't go back to the hospital, love. *Please*," I begged him.

"Crystal, we have to call and at least let them know what's going on!" He grabbed the discharge paperwork from my nightstand and walked out of the room. I could hear him speaking with someone and then the call ended. He returned and said, "Someone is going to call me back."

The doctor on call phoned and said, "Take her to Lenox Hill Hospital immediately. We've phoned ahead to notify them that you're coming." I clinched my eyes as I fought back a tear. The thought of going anywhere feeling like this was unfathomable. I'd been going into the city all week and I just wanted to rest in my bed.

Allen looked at me sternly. "We need to go."

I fought back. "Let's give it another hour, and if my fever goes down, I'll stay here."

"An hour is too long. I'll be back in 30 minutes to check your temperature again and if it hasn't gone down, we really need to go."

Thirty minutes went by and I was in and out of consciousness, falling asleep every few minutes. *I just want to sleep*, I thought, *I will feel much better in the morning.*

Thirty to forty minutes went by and Allen was back. I slid the thermometer under my tongue and within a minute it beeped. 102.6. I didn't feel bad at all. I was just cold and sleepy.

Allen started to raise his voice, "Either you take a cold shower or we're going!"

"Please don't be mad at me. I don't need that right now." It was difficult to explain how I felt. The thought of putting on clothes and going out into the chilled air to take an uncomfortable ride and wait in a hospital made me feel worse. Tears fell. "Please just give me another hour and if it's worse, I promise I'll go." I reflect now on this moment and how I felt. I was so at peace. I was comfortable and although cold, I was warm, and all I wanted was to fall asleep.

After some time, I turned my head to look at the clock: 30 minutes had passed. A small voice within said, *Get up and go now.* "Allen!"

He rushed in.

"I think I'm going to get dressed and go."

Without a word, Allen put on a hoodie and started getting dressed. I walked into my closet and found the big sweatpants I had worn when I had left the hospital 10 days ago. I bundled up in a full coat and scarf, and around 8 or 9p.m., Allen helped me to the elevator because I could barely stand or keep my eyes open. I felt extremely weak, with no fight left. The elevator doors opened and my eyes remained closed. I could only focus on putting one foot in front of the other. The doors opened and the chilled air hit my face; the sweat beads around my temple began to dry.

Allen helped me into the Uber. It was a nice black SUV with cushy seats with a Jamaican driver. I closed my eyes. I didn't see any city lights or tall buildings. I could only hear the conversation in the car but I just wanted to go to sleep. Ironically, the driver began to talk about how he'd never heard of Lenox Hill Hospital and that there were perfectly good hospitals in Brooklyn, but what you really need are herbs to keep you healthy and lots of juicing like "we do in Jamaica." He had no earthly idea what I was going through but was offering his advice anyway.

Allen's mom and dad are both from islands, so he and the driver had a
nice conversation. After what felt like an eternity, Allen said, "Open your eyes,
hun, we're here." Luckily, on that day in early May, there was barely anyone
in the emergency room. Allen pointed to the chairs and told me to take a
seat—he would sign me in. Wobbling, I found a seat at the very back corner
of the waiting area. I balled up and closed my eyes to sleep. Within a minute,
Allen returned. A wheelchair was brought over by a triage nurse. "We've been
expecting you for a few hours now. Come in so we can verify some information and check your vitals." I was wheeled into a triage-like area and pestered
with questions. The nurse and her assistant checked my blood pressure, heart
rate, and temperature.

The nurse checked my vitals again and began to look angry; her face was
scrounged up in confusion. She asked me, "Do you have sickle cell anemia?"

"No, never." She turned around and whispered something to the assistant
and took off in a full sprint. My vitals were topsy-turvy. My blood pressure was
deathly low. My temperature was nearing 104. My heart rate was through the
roof, as if I'd been running full speed through Central Park.

What happened next woke up every sense in my body.

The nurse tossed the paperwork on the desk and rolled me to the back
on two wheels. She yelled to Allen, "Stay here! Someone will come to get
you shortly. We need to get her back to the ER stat!" Within seconds I was
swarmed by a crew of nurses all sharing the information amongst each other.
They peeled off to get the appropriate tools with urgency. The next thing I
knew, I was levitating out of the wheelchair and there were multiple people

squeezing under my arms and legs to lift me onto a bed. The sense of urgency had me alarmed, terrified, and pain shot through my entire body. Someone said to me in the midst of the chaos, very loudly, "Ms. Brown? Can you hear me? Open your eyes, please. I know this is a lot, but your vitals are alerting us that we need to do a full panel of bloodwork on you to see what's going on, and since you recently underwent major surgery, we also need to complete a CAT scan. We need to get all of your clothes off now and get you changed. Do you understand?"

I closed my eyes and nodded my head.

The person nodded at the other parties in the room and they began to pull off my shoes, socks, pants, coat, sweater, bra, and undies. When they took my pants off, one nurse said, "We have a Foley! ...Were you released from the hospital with this Foley, Ms. Brown?"

I nodded my head and with a faint voice said, "It was replaced yesterday by a urologist."

"Okay, we need to remove it and replace it to make sure you have a new one since you're under our care now. Okay?"

I nodded. Tears emerged. Stickers were being placed all over my upper body for an EKG. My bed was raised so they could get a better look at the Foley. They removed all of the catheter accessories and took the tape off quickly. Two additional nurses were prepping a new Foley kit at the same time. The nurse who had placed the stickers received the vials for blood samples. Someone prepped one of my arms for blood work while the other arm was being cleaned with alcohol in preparation for an IV.

"You're going to feel a slight sting, okay, Ms. Brown?"

I nodded my head and looked away. The needle was in. After what felt like 10 vials of blood, the needle was removed. The IV was now in the other arm and fluids were started. The catheter went in with ease. I was finally fully covered with a hospital gown and blanket. I continued to convulse and shiver.

"Ms. Brown, we'll be back shortly. We have someone coming to bring you fluids to drink in preparation for the CAT scan. It's very important that you drink all of the fluids as quickly as you can, so we can get you upstairs for a scan. We are running the blood work now to rule things out and get more clues as to what's going on, okay?"

"Okay, thank you," I mustered.

For a few minutes, all went quiet. I didn't know how much time had passed because it felt like a tornado of activity all centered around my body. I pushed my head further into the pillow. I couldn't believe I was back in there. What could possibly be wrong? *I'm just sleepy and cold*, I told myself. I closed my eyes and within a few minutes someone brought Allen back to the room and handed him the bag with my clothes. "We will keep you both updated. You'll need to stay the night, so we're working on a room for you now. After the CAT scan, you'll be released to a room." Standing right behind the nurse was another woman with different scrubs who brought in the fluid I needed to drink. She handed me a cup and gave me the instructions. I drank the first cup while she was in the room. She asked, "Do you need anything?"

"Another blanket, please."

"Let me ask." She returned and said, "Ms. Brown, the team needs to get your fever down, so they aren't going to give you another blanket right now. I'm so sorry."

I pursed my lips and nodded. The liquid was cold and I felt like ice. I didn't want to drink that stuff. I didn't have any room in my belly. My stomach felt like stone inside and the last thing I wanted was to lie there and drink that.

I closed my eyes again.

Allen said, "Come on, you have to drink it."

I rolled my eyes toward the opposite curtain and took a deep breath. I didn't feel like fighting. I just wanted to lie there. After some coaching from Allen, I sat up and drank the liquid. Every few minutes, another cup. Cup after cup, and after some time I got all of the fluid down. Then we waited.

The head ER doctor called Allen outside to talk with him privately. They both came back in and some news was shared, but I kept fading in and out of consciousness. Something about sepsis. *Sepsis!* I woke up to listen. "Ms. Brown, if you had not come in when you did, you could have suffered from septic shock, which can be fatal. You did the right thing. Someone will be down within an hour to take you up for the CAT scan. We have more information now, but we need to see what else is going on. We also need to do a rectal scan and capture images as well. This will happen at the same time as your CAT scan. I know you don't feel great, but we're here to help."

"Thank you," I said. I was in shock.

Now, we waited. The time was about 11p.m. I heard one man screaming in agony: "When is someone going to come in here and see about me!"

"Sir, we're going to treat you, but you should consider speaking with someone about substance abuse. Do you have somewhere you can go when we release you?"

"No, I was kicked out."

"Okay, well, we will give you the names of some places."

From the bit I could hear through the curtain, he'd fallen down at a bar and had been knocked unconscious. Allen told me there was a gunshot wound victim hanging outside my curtained off area waiting for a room. He had been shot in the Bronx. I don't know how medical professionals are able to deal with this sort of stuff. They are the real heroes. I tried to tune it all out and rest my eyes.

Around midnight, someone came in and said, "I'm here to take you up for your CAT scan." He pressed buttons on the bed and suddenly I was mobile. The bed rolled and we were off. Getting out of the ER was a bit of a blur, with lots of noises, bright lights, and voices. We took the elevator up to the floor where the scan would be performed. In the room, there were several CAT scan doctors and staff, plus one of the colorectal surgery residents I recognized from my round one stay in the hospital. They all greeted me and said, "We're going to lift you up and place you on the table here. Ready? Okay, on the count of 3... 1,2,3 slide." They slid me over to the table and gave me a pillow. After a blur of instructions, everyone left the room and they started the process. I glided down into the machine and they got the footage they needed. Before I came out, the colorectal resident told me, "I know they told you already downstairs, but we need to grab images of the inside of the rectum where the rectal resection was performed to make sure the fuse is secure and there aren't any holes. In order to do this, I have a small catheter and I'm going to inject contrast into your bottom in order to light up the rectal area so we can get a good solid picture of what's going on. I know you're not excited about this, but I promise to make it as comfortable as I can. You will feel a little pressure but there shouldn't be any pain." I trusted her. She was nice and thorough with her explanations. She walked me through every step. "I'm going to lift your gown now. Bring your bottom a little further down. Okay, I'm going to insert the catheter now so you'll feel some light pressure, but you shouldn't feel any pain. Are you in pain?"

"No, I'm not in pain."

"I'm going to insert the contrast now and we'll start the scan."

Suddenly, I felt cold liquid flowing through my rectal cavity. It was not the most pleasant thing I'd been through, but definitely not the worst. I heard the machine capturing the images.

"Okay, Ms. Brown, all done. I'm removing the catheter now and I'm going to wipe up some of the liquid here. I'll place a pad under your bottom to absorb the liquid."

I thanked her for being there and making me feel comfortable.

"No problem at all. You've been through a lot. Let us know if you need anything. We're going to take a look at the images and the team will determine next steps. You get to go to your room now."

Someone rolled me onto another floor and into my hospital room. My nurse welcomed me to the room and said, "I'll be back shortly to get your vitals."

At that point, I was in and out again. Sometime later, the nurse, doctor, and staff walked into the room to give me more news. "Ms. Brown, we've located a DVT (a blood clot) and abscess cavity in your pelvic area. There is a tiny hole in the place where your rectum was fused back together, and because it was not completely sealed, it has created an abscess cavity about the size of a grapefruit and we need to get it drained as quickly as possible. We are still reviewing the DVT to determine the best course of action here. We may need to operate again and place a filter in your pelvic cavity, but with the abscess and recent surgery, it is very risky. Right now, we are going to start a Heparin drip intravenously. We'll need to add another IV to the opposite arm, as nothing else but the blood thinner can be placed on that side of the body. We need to treat the abscess cavity immediately. We've already called in the IR (Interventional Radiology) doctor—Dr. Gill—here at Lenox Hill. He's on his way, and as soon as he arrives, we will need to get you prepped for IR surgery. We are leaving you on NPO (nothing by mouth) in the meantime. We need to get this under control as timely as possible."

The doctor pointed to my legs and directed the nurse to put floaties on my legs (compression sleeves). She left the room to retrieve them. I complied to everything and Allen thanked everyone for the updates and attention. He asked a couple of questions and I closed my eyes again. It was a lot to take in. I had no idea what was next, but it didn't sound like I would be resting anytime soon.

The nurse returned and prepped my other arm for an IV. I felt like I was on a cross being crucified. Both hands were tied down with IVs. The Heparin drip was started. The nurse warned me that I would likely need another IV for other meds, so I would have three in total. One for the blood thinner. One for fluids intravenously. And another for meds. *Wonderful.* I rested my eyes for a bit, but before I could doze off, the doors flew open, and we were off again.

Dr. Gill had arrived and was being prepped for the procedure. I was wheeled off to a quiet floor, where I lay on my hospital bed in the hall. I looked around for a clock: 2a.m. The doctor came out and went over the diagnosis with Allen and I again and explained that he was going to place a needle and drain into my bottom to drain the fluid. The fluid would seep out into a bulb that I would be given instructions on how to care for. He gave me a paper to sign and we were off. I squeezed Allen's hand and we slowly let go as I was carried away. The doctor wheeled me right into the operation room and there were four or five of us in total. His team prepped me and slid me over from my hospital bed to the operating table. They gave me a pillow and blanket to cover my lower legs and explained that I would be under light anesthesia for the procedure because there would be a bit of pain. They needed to create an entry point in my bottom for the JP drain. Through glossy eyes I nodded, in a daze.

After a few minutes, the doctor was ready to begin. The nurse covered my face with the gas and told me to take a few deep breaths. Within seconds, everything went dark.

I woke up and realized I was back on my hospital bed outside the room.

"How are you feeling?" the doctor asked.

I managed to respond with one word: "Pain."

"I'll make sure the nurse gives you some pain meds through your IV."

A tear dripped down one side of my face.

The doctor chatted with Allen while I bobbled between earthside and the unknown. I didn't know how much more I could take. I was lying on my side. Something felt foreign. I patted myself and tapped around my left butt cheek. There was a long tube sticking out. I felt my way down to the end and saw a bulb. I felt empty and confused. *God, please help me.* I closed my eyes and fell asleep.

After a few hours, a nurse entered the dark hospital room to check my vitals. I could hear Allen sleeping. She asked if I needed anything and left as quickly as she had came. That happened every couple of hours. I opened my eyes again and realized I'd made it to morning. I couldn't have anything to eat still, so I just lay in the bed with my thoughts. I could feel myself sinking into self-pity.

Sunday. Around 7a.m., the on-call doctor stopped in to speak with us. He pushed around on my belly and checked the new tube. After the doctor left, Allen explained everything to me: "Crystal, I'm not going to lie, last night was rough. The ER staff said that if we hadn't gotten you to the hospital, it's doubtful you could've survived the night without medical attention. Now, you have to have this tube in to help drain the abscess and it needs to stay in until the fluid is gone and the hole in your rectum is fully healed."

I took a deep breath and sighed it out. I let his words sink in as we sat in silence.

Soon after, one of the CNAs came in to empty my catheter bag and measure the urine output. A wave of embarrassment came over me but there was nothing I could do. I looked away and thanked the nurse. Then, for the first time since we had arrived, I was alone. (Allen had left to get breakfast for himself.) I lay on my side and I sank deeply into the pillows. I mentally bounced back and forth between listening to the steady hum of activity outside the room, and the morning NYC buzz outside on the street, until the next nurse visited. No one could tell me when I would be going home, so I began to watch the sun and shadows on the building outside. I could barely move and I didn't want to.

Now that I could rest, I realized that if Allen had not been there, if he'd gone to PA to visit family, I would be dead. Like *dead-dead*. I would have certainly never thought to check my temperature. Never thought to call the doctor. Never gone to Lenox Hill's emergency room. I would have slept the night and woken in Heaven. Endo was feeling more and more like a death sentence with each passing day. I welled up with emotion all over again. *When will the tears stop?* I'd cried enough tears in the past twelve months to fill the Atlantic Ocean. "Thank you" was all I can manage to say when Allen returned.

11

DEFEATED

N ow it was Monday. I woke up attempting to adjust to my new normal. I didn't want to do anything but sleep and dream because dreams were far better than my reality. My stomach was a brick wall and I needed to lie on my side. Around 6:30a.m., the hum in the hallways began to pick up as doctors and residents made their morning rounds. The first group to see me each morning was Gynecology. They discussed my medical history, diagnosis, and current status outside of the door before walking in.

"Good morning, Ms. Brown, how are you feeling today?"

"Okay," I said.

"I'm going to take a look at you," the doctor said. She put on her gloves and pulled up my hospital gown to press on my abdomen. All of the residents leaned in to take a look at what she was doing and how.

"We will be by to check on you tomorrow, okay? Take care."

The GYN crew left—on to the next hospital patient. Within minutes, the Colorectal residents stopped in to check on me as well.

"Any bowel movements yet? I'm assuming no, but have to ask."

"No, not yet." They left. I imagined them going to the next patient.

The next set of visitors usually included one of my actual surgeons, Vascular, IR, and either Dr. Le, Dr. Ari, or both. They stopped in to ask how I was doing and I told them about the spasms and the hardness of my belly.

"It will improve, but it's important to get moving as soon as you can. The more movement, the better."

After the morning visits, the CNA came by to check my vitals again. Shortly after that, Phlebotomy came by to take a sample of blood. Vitals were checked and blood was drawn every few hours. My room felt cold. It was oddly quiet on that side of the floor. I was in a corner, so there wasn't much foot traffic. Allen came by in the evening to check on me. I told him how hard it was to rest because of all the visitors each hour. He stayed with me for about an hour, until nearly 10p.m.

Tuesday. The next day. Day 4. After morning visits were over, my nurse came by. "I heard about your stomach. I'm going to give you an extra dose of Colace this morning. Do you want to go for a walk today?"

I thought I should. I was finally feeling stable enough to try.

"Make sure you're doing your breathing, too, while you're lying in bed."

"Okay," I told her. I lay in bed and stared at the whiteboard. I hadn't had anything to eat in three days. I stared at my hands and made a fist. One of the IVs had a bit of blood around it and I internalized what I saw. My entire situation felt like such a mess. I couldn't eat, sleep much, or pee. All I could see were limitations. I fought with myself about getting up to walk. I knew I should, but my body didn't want to. I tested the sturdiness of my bed by tugging at it a little. I pushed the button to sit up and lowered the base of the bed so my feet were closer to the ground. One leg at a time, I removed the compression sleeves. I stared up at the wires and figured out which lines went to which arms. I finally lifted myself up to a seated position and took a deep breath. Next were my legs. I needed to get one leg at a time over the edge and secure the bags around each leg. I got the right leg over, then reached to grab my left calf muscle, but the IV line stopped me. I had two IVs on the right and one on the left for the Heparin drip. I moved the lines around to give myself more freedom and guided my left leg over the edge. I sat for some time and finally pushed just enough to get both feet on the ground. Inch by inch, I stood. My back throbbed from bad posture, muscle atrophy, and resting in the same spot for days and days. I tied the back of my gown as best I could and used the nurse's station to lean on. I made it out to the door, down the hall a bit, and back. That completed my activity for the day.

Allen called to ask how I was doing. "Any better?" My family told me I needed prune juice, so I asked the night nurse to bring some. Doctors came in throughout the day from various departments. Vascular came by. "Hey Ms. Brown, have you experienced any swelling since you've arrived?"

"No."

"Okay, we've decided it's best that we don't perform any new operations on you right now. We are going to keep you on Heparin and keep a close eye on you for the next few days." That was such a relief. (I sent Allen and mom a message to share the good news. One less surgery!) They were also thinking about sending me home the next day and putting me on the pill form of blood thinners.

Wednesday. I woke up feeling terrible. My stomach was beginning to swell and I hadn't had a bowel movement in over a week. I was fatigued from not having eaten. I sent Allen a note:

Please bring me some real prune juice. The one they brought me is mostly sugar. I'm tired of Ensure and water.

Okay, I will. Make sure you get up and go for a walk again.

Thursday. The main gynecological surgeon stopped by to check on me. He told me he knew I was disappointed and frustrated about all of this, but endometriosis is a silent but ravaging disease that tears women apart. He proceeded to tell me horror stories about women who also had stage 4 endo, who had feces and urine coming out of places they shouldn't. I interpreted that as his way of saying *suck it up and persevere because you must*. Oddly, I did feel better hearing those gut-wrenching stories. Maybe my situation wasn't so bad. When he left, though, I cried. I cried for the women who had it worse than I did. His words were somewhat tormenting because I felt my own pain was being diminished, but it was also a good pep talk. I was emotionally exhausted.

Allen asked if I wanted to get up and walk. I just didn't have it in me. I had to sleep on my side now because the drain was there, always there. I drifted off without a fight.

Friday. Day 6. The medical team made the morning rounds and everyday my news was the same: my stomach hurt and it hurt to walk or move. That day, however, something new happened: I was able to go to the bathroom in the night and had had a bowel movement. The team told me this was positive and it meant my body was fighting to course correct and I should be able to begin eating solids again. They added notes to my chart and left the room. Shortly after, a nurse told me I would be able to have lunch or dinner that day, and that was usually a good sign: if all went well, I could go home the next day. "They want to keep an eye on you to make sure you don't get sick after eating," she said. The lunchroom lady came by with a menu. After nearly six days, I could eat. I put in my order for lunch and, for the first time in a while, I was excited about something. That something wasn't a cute handbag or boots, but a hospital cafeteria meal. I ordered the chicken dish with mashed potatoes and carrots. I wasn't very hungry after going without eating for so long, but I was excited about eating again, which told me I was making progress.

The food came and Allen snapped a photo of me for posterity and as proof to our family that I was one major step closer to being released. I rolled to my side and ate away. Later, the nurse checked on me. I told her everything was fine. I ate and felt a rush of energy I desperately needed. I "walked" around my room a bit with the fluids, and with the nurse's station as a walker.

Saturday. Day 7. The day finally arrived. After seven excruciating and exhausting days, I could finally go home! Allen arrived after work and was pleasantly surprised by my demeanor. I was sitting up in bed smiling. I couldn't wait to use my own shower and lie in my own bed! I was eager for the nurse's update. She said, "It won't be long now before I can begin processing your discharge paperwork. Since you've been back on solid foods, you haven't had any issues, and you're going to the bathroom without major issues."

Allen had a bag with clothes for me to wear home. After what seemed like hours, the nurse told me discharge is underway! I was going home, but thinking about those at the hospital, who weren't so lucky, tempered my excitement.

Someone came in to go over the discharge instructions with me, which included all of the meds I needed to take: pain meds; antibiotics; Colace; and now, Eliquis. I acknowledged and signed the papers. I was free! Allen put my supplies into a few bags and headed downstairs to meet his uncle, who had offered to take us home from the hospital again. I waited on the side of the bed in silence, looking around the room and breathing a sigh of relief. *I'm going to live.*

A guy with a Bronx accent showed up with a wheelchair to roll me outside. I gingerly stood up. My legs felt like pencils. I'd lost so much weight. I eased down into the chair breathing heavily. I sat on one side of the wheelchair because my drain wouldn't allow me to sit comfortably anymore.

"I'm ready," I told him.

"Let's get you out of here."

I smiled and nodded. I told the nursing staff thank you on my way out and they told me to hang in there and take good care. I acknowledged them with a head nod. As I was wheeled into the elevator, I took it all in. I had a feeling I won't be back there anytime soon.

On Level 1, I was gently wheeled over bumps as I held my stomach and balanced on one leg. Everything still hurt, but the sheer joy of leaving impeded the pain signals in my brain. Within seconds, I was in the cool crisp air again. I eased out of the chair, into the back seat of the car, and we were off. I looked back at Lenox Hill until we bended the corner.

I stared out of the window. I felt better as I looked out at the city lights and the pedestrians walking, running, living. We glided over the Brooklyn Bridge and, before we knew it, we were home.

The doormen welcomed me back and I nodded and waved as I eased my way to the elevator. By the time we got into our apartment, I felt fatigue creep in. I had to take a real shower first though. I hadn't showered since I had left for the hospital a week ago. I sat in the bathroom for a minute before taking off my clothes and looking at myself in the mirror. I didn't recognize the woman staring back. I extended my arms and looked at the needle prick holes beginning to scab, and bruises on my arms and hands. I looked at the three IV sites. I looked at the Foley bag on my right leg and my latest fashion accessory: the JP drain tube and bulb hanging and strapped around my left leg.

I eased into the shower, held on to the side, and let the water wash away the last week. I tucked the JP bulb into the strap on my leg and leaned against the wall. After a good scrub, I lay in the bed. I was starting from zero. My fever had crept up just from travelling from the hospital to our apartment. Allen gave me my meds and put the Deontay Wilder fight on. The fight night was at Barclays, just down the street from us. We had made plans to go to see it a few months back but hadn't bought tickets, thankfully. Wilder knocked down his opponent in 137 seconds. I was home now; time to rebuild for my own fight.

I spent the next week lying in bed, only getting up in the morning to complete my usual routine and lie back down. I wake up every few hours to the prescribed meds on my discharge paperwork. I had a banana or orange around noon to serve as breakfast and lunch. I wasn't in the mood to eat much. I forced myself to clean a little bit each day, but only managed being on my feet for a few minutes before getting winded. My mom sent flowers and I stared at them between dozing in and out all day. Allen caught an earlier train home that week to check on me. I was beginning to hate sitting near him. The smell of the fluid seeping through the tube of the JP drain was awful. I smelled like I was rotting, like a moldy piece of old fruit.

On Friday, I woke and looked at the drain. I squeezed the tube and looked at the bulb. It had blood and fluids sloshing around in it. It was getting full, so I needed to get up, measure the contents, and empty it out. My stomach turned at the sight of it. I held onto the tube as I walked to the bathroom. I grabbed a glove, pried the bulb open, and poured the contents into a small container I had been given in my hospital bag on the day of my discharge. I squeezed the bulb and a dull ache crept into my left side as I reclosed it. I slid off the glove and wrote down the amount of the contents, poured it into the toilet, and flushed. I was disgusted with myself. I avoided looking up into the mirror. I retreated to bed.

Saturday now. Saturday used to be my favorite day of the week. I used to get up early to go for a run while the city was sleeping. Allen would grab breakfast from a bodega and we'd eat, read, and rest a while until we picked a spot to eat for lunch. Now, I was sitting in the apartment, covering up the drain with a blanket, hoping the smell won't seep through to Allen. I could smell it and it didn't go away. I was so self-conscious, I could barely eat. Allen sat near me and I yelled at him to move down to the end of the couch. He said, "Stop it, I don't care. You're making a big deal out of this."

"It *is* a big deal," I screamed back. "You don't understand!"

"Alright, whatever."

I covered my face and sank into the couch on my one good side. I sat on the couch half the day—an improvement from staying in bed all day.

That night, I pretended to climb into bed until Allen was asleep, then I hobbled to the couch and covered myself with some blankets. I lay on my right with my left side pointing upward. Nothing could touch the JP drain site without me wincing. It had been a week and my neck was slowly getting a crook from my only using one side of my body to rest on. I had tried lying on my back and it had hurt so badly. I couldn't lie on my stomach because the incisions hurt. I couldn't sleep well, so I dozed in and out all day. I hadn't gotten over the trauma from surgery and now I was dealing with the fact that I could've and maybe should've died last Saturday.

My thoughts spiraled into the deep, where I had sworn to never go again. I smelled like death. *Maybe I should be dead.* As tears trickled down my face to my right hand as it supported my head, I didn't wipe them. I let them come furiously until I began to wail. *Why God? You should have let me go. I smell like death… I should be dead…* I kept repeating that as my hands began to shake. *Why am I here?*

I need you to live, a still, small voice said.

I grew silent a while. I cried harder. Why was God talking to me after what I'd been through?

Allen heard me and came out of the room. "What are you doing out here? It's cold out here. You're shaking."

"Don't come any closer. I smell like death." I could barely get the words out without losing my breath. I wept even harder. "Stay away from me. I smell like death. I can't sleep. I smell like death. I can smell death."

Allen grabbed my hand with both of his and closed his eyes. "You'll get through this, Crystal. Let me get you some tissue." He returned with a box of tissues for me to blow my nose and wipe my face. I told him to go back to bed, that I would be fine. I continued to shake until I realized I was still alive. I reached over the edge of the couch for my phone and began to play the same song I had played the night Welan had violated me. I listened to the song over and over until my body began to calm down. *Pull yourself out of the deep. I need you to live*, God said. *I need you to live.*

On Sunday, I felt better. I was still embarrassed about the smell, but realized it was temporary. Allen left to go to visit his mom with his uncle and grandma. I decided to find some real clothes to put on and go for a walk. I found my big sweats and a hoodie. It was 70-plus degrees outside, but I didn't care; I needed to stay warm. I grabbed my cane and walked around the floor of our apartment a few times. Then I made breakfast. *I must keep living*, I told myself.

When Allen returned, he looked refreshed and happy. His mom had made a soup; and his grandmother, her famous fish cakes and some vegetable sides. "They made this stuff just for you," he said, "My grandma is still downstairs if you're up for walking outside to see them."

Allen held my arm and I held the wall as we made our way downstairs. I leaned against the corner of the elevator and caught my breath. When the door slid open, I tried to stand a bit taller.

The air was crisp, refreshing, but made me feel vulnerable: I hadn't been outside in a week. We walked up to the car and Allen's 90-year-old grandmother got out, gave me a tight squeeze, and said, "I've been praying for you. Everything is going to work out just fine. Don't worry. I hope you guys enjoy the food. You can't stay out here long, but it's good to see you. You're looking good. You're going to get strong. Watch. Don't worry yourself one bit." I smiled bigger than I had in a while. She understood. I give her one last hug, hugged Uncle Ray, and thanked them both again. We went back upstairs to heat up the food. The food was just what I needed.

The next week I was determined to get out of bed at a reasonable time and find things to do. My mom had brought a care package for me during the first surgery, so I decided to open the hospital bag and find it. Inside were books, puzzles, and mazes. I decided to start tackling the 500-piece puzzle one piece at a time.

I had to visit Dr. Roberts' office. Begrudgingly, I attempted taking the train into the city. I watched an older woman get off the train and ease her way across the platform to get the local. I saw her frailty amongst the crowded station, with people zipping around her like a swarm of bees. I followed her lead and waited for my next train. After seeing Roberts and hearing the same story again—that "it will come back, give it time"—he sent me out the door with a prescription for the UTI I thought I had from the catheter. I looked at my phone to check the time. Barely any time had passed between my arrival and then. I was feeling isolated and frustrated, not knowing if I should cry or be angry. Who was there to be angry at? I decided to clear my head and take a walk. What could I do besides go back to the same apartment with the same four walls? I could stress eat. That would fix it. I ran choices through my mind and settled on cupcakes. I pulled up one of my favorite bakeries through the phone's GPS and realized it was a 1-mile walk. I was determined to do it. If I could run a marathon, I could walk. I walk to clear my head and I needed this desperately. I remembered the woman on the train. The invisibility of the frail.

I watched the birds on the sidewalk and the squirrels in the trees as I went by. I thought of the wealth in that neighborhood. I smiled at the people who made an effort to make eye contact. Some blocks were full of life; others were silent. On the silent blocks, I found rest by leaning against a wall or sitting on a stoop, if only for a brief moment. After what felt like an eternity, I made it to the bakery. The air was cool as I opened the door and I had the little store to myself. I told the associate what I wanted in my mix and she boxed it up for me. I'd done it. I'd completed the mile, though it had taken me an hour and it should have been 15-20 minutes max.

Outside, I stood until the traffic light changed twice. There was a Lush store across the way. I was getting closer to shops I liked. I decided to go into Lush to look around and then catch the train home. I gathered enough courage and energy to cross the street, just barely making it before the light turned green again. I entered the store with sweat beads running down my back. I was barely inside when my legs collapsed beneath me. I was on the ground. I heard someone call for help and one of the store associates ran to me and asked, "Are you okay?"

"Yes, I'm fine."

They helped me to my feet and I leaned against the checkout stand. I was mortified.

Someone grabbed a chair and I reached up to hold the side of it for stability and pulled myself up. Embarrassed, I sat without looking anyone in the eyes. The same associate scurried to bring a cup of water to me. "Do you need an ambulance?"

"No, no, please no."

"Can I call someone for you?"

"No, thank you. Seriously, I'm okay. I just need to go home. I'll call an Uber." I hung my head in shame. I sipped the water another few minutes and left the store with my head still tilted downward. Several people walked me to the door and helped me out. They stared for a bit until I got to the corner. I could feel the eyes on my back. I turned and waved thanks. Completely out of fuel, I crossed one more street and, in the middle of the next block (where no one who saw the fall could see me), I leaned against a building, with labored breathing, and hailed a ride through my phone. I was embarrassed, disappointed, and frustrated with my body. I placed a pin for the end of the block, away from the incident. Within a minute, an Uber arrived. I gripped the door handle and bent over to ease my way into the car. I sat on the one butt cheek

I could use and, for the first time in a while, I didn't look out the window. I closed my eyes wishing the world would disappear.

I was in a melancholy mood for the rest of the day. At home, I placed the cupcakes on the counter. I didn't want them anymore. *What's the point of it all?* I thought. I mustered up enough energy to shower and climb back into bed.

I worked on the puzzle more the next day, a little longer every day. I was able to work on it for about an hour before getting too tired. It was nice to have something to do besides watching TV and reading books all day.

On Thursday, I got dressed to see Dr. Ari again for my follow-up post-ER visit. I caught a cab to take me to Midtown. I sat in the back and watched the buildings shine and glisten. In Dr. Ari's office, he checked the JP drain site, the tube, and the bulb, and asked how much fluid was coming out on average, and how I was feeling overall. "I've been better," I told to him, "I'm still having some accidents with my bowels." He started to say *we had to go so deep to remove the nodule and there were some risks* and I gave him a look like, *sure, this isn't making me feel better, so please let's end this part of our chat.* I asked him, "How long will I need the JP drain?"

"We will have to play it by ear, but at least another three weeks. When do you see Dr. Gill again? Okay, I want you to come back and see me then as well."

The visit was brief. I headed back home and lay down.

The next day, I woke, made breakfast, and started on my puzzle. I was about 75% done. I played some music, got started, and didn't finish until the sun began to go down. It was the weekend again—time to have some fun! Saturday morning, I asked Allen to take me on a walk. We made our way to the outdoor space in our building, sat for some time, caught up on current events, and talked about what had been going on at work. Back in our apartment, we ordered takeout from our favorite Brooklyn restaurant and binged shows for the rest of the day. The weekend was always a much-needed distraction from the reality of my situation.

Monday again. It was now June. In New York, we were heading into festival and outdoor activity season. I began to realize that it had been over a month since my surgery and all the events I'd planned to go to, I needed to cancel. A festival on Governor's Island—cancelled. My grandmother's surprise 90th birthday party in Alabama—cancelled. A friend's baby shower in New Jersey— cancelled. As the days and minutes passed, I looked at social media to see what I'd missed: all the fun videos and pictures of friends enjoying priceless moments. My grandmother's 90th birthday party hit me the hardest. I called my mom. She said, "Hey, I'm getting ready to head over to Alabama for the party. I need to pick up cups and plates for everyone before I get there."

"Well, have fun. Can you please send me pictures tonight afterward? I really hate I'm missing it."

"That's alright. You're right where you should be, dear. Your Grandma understands. I'll call you later."

My mom sent the photos that night and, in the darkness of the room, my face lit up with a smile and watery eyes. Most of my family was there and my grandmother looked so happy. *I missed it all.* My smile began to hurt from keeping tears away.

The next Monday, I woke up and out of habit reached for the cane, then realized, it was time to chuck it. My abdomen was slowly waking up and I could now move without feeling like I would tear a hole in my incisions. I'd figured out how to safety pin the JP drain to the side of my left leg and keep the Foley bag on the right side of my right leg. I followed my normal morning routine, but added a morning and afternoon walk around the building. I walked my floor, then hit the elevator to walk around different floors, so people wouldn't think I was weird or trying to break in. I planned to make my way outside by the end of the week. I was feeling pretty good.

By Thursday, I was itching to get outside and go somewhere.

"Why don't we go to the movies?" Allen suggested. "You think you're up for it? ...I'll get the tickets."

I was so excited on Friday. I put on two hoodies and my big pants and tucked my wallet and keys into my pocket. With my hands in my pockets (to hold up the bags on my legs and the makeshift harnesses), I walked toward the Target that was one block away. Inside, I held the escalator rail tight. I made my way to the women's clothing section. I wanted something nice to wear to the movies and those big sweatpants weren't it. I walked around and found a cute dress—wide and long enough to hide my bags. As I made my way to check out, I spotted a black halter jumper. I looked to see if they had one my size—they did. I put back the dress and smiled inside. I was going on a date tomorrow after weeks of hospitals, doctors' appointments, and staring at the four walls in my apartment!

12

GLIMMER OF HOPE

Saturday afternoon, I took my time and got dressed up for the first time in a very long time. I didn't care about the bags and bulbs around my legs. I didn't have any cares for a change and that was a nice feeling. We hit a matinee at a theatre close by. Walking back home was a little challenging, but I didn't feel much pain in my body.

On Sunday, we made breakfast and enjoyed talking to family and relaxing. It had been a while. I was genuinely smiling. We found a new show to binge and eventually drifted off to sleep with the window open, listening to the sound of Brooklyn as we rested easy for a change.

Monday was a big day. I needed to go back to the hospital so Dr. Gill from the IR team could look at the JP drain and see if it could be removed today! I was so hopeful and nervous, I didn't know what to do. Allen decided to work from home for half the day so he could go with me. The last time I had gone into IR, I had come out fuzzy, in agonizing pain, with a tube sticking out of my bottom. We stepped into the city air. People were buzzing about on their phones heading to work.

"I'll call an Uber for us," Allen said.

"No, let's take the train up. I can do it."

"Okay," he replied, with a surprised look. As we waited for the train, the rush of the warm air as the train arrived made me feel alive again. I sat in the first seat I saw and braced myself, sitting forward so the drain wouldn't rub against the seat. When we reached 77th Street, I took my time with one hand on the rail and one hand on Allen's shoulder, one step at a time. At the hospital, we got our IDs scanned and we signed in.

IR was expecting me, so I get scooted straight back to the room I had been in almost one month ago, where the IR nurses were ready to prep me. "Hey, Ms. Brown, we are going to get you prepped for Dr. Gill. He will check the JP drain and push fluid through the tube to see if there is still a leak at the resection site. If there is no leak, we will go ahead and remove the tube."

"Will I need to be under anesthesia again?"

"No, not this time. It should be pretty painless. You may feel a bit of pressure is all... Go ahead and lie down here and make yourself comfortable. Let us know if you need another pillow... I'm going to pull your pants down back here to expose this one side so Dr. Gill can see, okay?"

Dr. Gill walked in. "Ms. Brown, how have you been feeling? How's the drainage?"

"I don't know. It was draining a lot, but it's slowing down and the tube itself appears mucky."

"Okay, let me take a look... Yeah, I see what you mean. I'm going to open this up and inject some fluid into the tube because I want to get a visual of the abscess and see if there is still a leak. Even a small leak could cause catastrophic damage... Fluid is going in now."

I felt pressure but no pain, until suddenly it felt as if someone had blown air into my butt cheek.

"You doing okay?" asked Dr. Gill.

"Yes," I managed to get out. I winced with my eyes closed. One of the nurses looked at me like a wounded puppy, but didn't speak. I held my breath as the doctor asked me to stay as still as possible.

"Almost there... There was a bit of a blockage. The fluid is in... Okay, we're done.... Well, Crystal, unfortunately there is still a leak and we won't be able to remove the drain today. We need to keep it in for now. I'll let Dr. Ari know."

I suddenly felt weak. Dr. Gill replaced the gauze and tape that kept the needle to the abscess in place on my cheek. The nurse helped me to my feet and Dr. Gill was gone before I could say goodbye. "Okay, Ms. Brown, you are free to go. We will alert Dr. Ari and you will follow up with his office going forward. If he wants you to come back here, he will let us know. Best of luck to you."

My forehead felt heavy and hot. Allen was waiting for me outside the door. I shook my head, signaling to him that no, the tube was still in. In the elevator back down to the lobby I closed my eyes. My head felt light and my muscles weak. Allen was on a work call and on the other line with his sister Rena. We stood outside for a few minutes and it began to rain softly. I grabbed a rail and tried to lean back against it. My stomach was churning now and my mouth began to water. I gripped the rail with my hands and before I knew it, I was on the ground vomiting.

"Rena, Rena, let me call you back," I heard Allen say. "What's going on? What happened?"

"I don't know... I can't move... I can't move." I think the tube had been blocked and they'd pushed the abscess fluid around when unblocking the tube. I vomited again until my ribs hurt. People passed by, peeking down from under their umbrellas. They walked around me.

"Here," Allen said, handing me a napkin he had found in his laptop bag.

"I need to go back to IR," I managed to get out, "I don't know what's wrong with me."

We went back up to Interventional Radiology and Allen told the nurses what had happened. They held my arms and took me to what appeared to be a recovery or waiting room. I was covered in sweat and rain. I cannot imagine what I looked like to those people and I didn't care.

"Here's some water, Ms. Brown, and a pill for the nausea. We can send some nausea pills/patches to your pharmacy and give you a few to take with you before you go. I'm sorry this is happening to you."

Allen had to leave for work. He said, "Let me know when you're home. I'll call you later to check in." I nodded through glazed eyes.

I sat with my eyes closed, hoping and praying the room would stop spinning. After thirty minutes or so, it did. "I think I'm okay now," I told them. With shaky hands, chills, and sweat beading on my temples, I inched my way out of the chair and back down the elevator, straight into an Uber, and home.

Back home, I managed to shower and climb into bed. I couldn't sleep

because of the pain, but I closed my eyes—hours and hours passed by. I got a
call from Dr. Le asking me how I was doing. "The drain and Foley are still in."

"Okay. Let's get you on the schedule. I want to see you in the office."

I really appreciated her going above and beyond this entire time. She was
the most empathetic doctor I'd ever met. I lay in bed for the next day and
a half. I didn't move because it aroused pain and nausea. I was angry now.
Not sad or frustrated, just angry. Angry because I had been getting better and
beginning to heal, and now I couldn't move without pain and discomfort.
I lay in bed for the next seven days, the only exceptions being vomiting and
diarrhea and the occasional snack. I was angry at the world. My stomach was
knotted up and I was on pain meds again. Some days I didn't eat at all. Some
days I didn't sleep. The abscess was angry and so was I.

For the rest of the week and weekend, I lay in bed feeling hopeless. Allen was out of town that weekend so I stayed in pajamas all day. My stomach
felt like concrete again. I was fighting off a fever daily and I didn't have an
appetite. I didn't want to do anything but lie there and sink deeper into the
bed. I sat in bed and cancelled my flight to Atlanta. A tear rolled down my
cheek to my ear, and then the pillow. I stared at the spot and closed my eyes.
Days began to run together and, one by one, I began to cancel more plans and
social activities. Allen told me I needed to get up and move around. I rolled
my eyes at him and ignored his words. I was not doing anything. I oscillated
between reading books and watching television for the next week until I had
to get up again.

Ten days later, I was finally forced out of bed. More doctor appointments. The blood clot they had found in my leg needed to be checked out. I made my way back to the hospital. When I got out of the car and onto the sidewalk, I stared at the ground I had been clutching just ten days ago. I walked into the hospital and this time they told me I was in the wrong area. I needed to go back out of the doors and enter from the Emergency Room doors and make the first left. I'd been to the ER there before as well, so I'd become well acquainted with the building and its nooks and crannies. I entered the elevator. There was a lovely older gentleman making jokes and it brightened my mood for the first time in a while. *People need people, Crystal*, I thought to myself. I'd isolated myself from everyone. Those who are hurting the most are the ones who need others the most. I stepped onto the Vascular floor and stood in line to get checked in. Every single patient in the waiting room was older than sixty. Some sat with caregivers. Others, with their partners. Others sat alone. It was a full house and I was the outlier.

After some time, my name was called and I was taken to a room to have my vitals checked. I was told to sit tight, that someone would be in soon to grab images. A young professional nurse came in after some time and was surprised to see someone my age. We chatted as she prepped me for the ultrasound. She wanted to see if she could find the blood clot in my left leg. As she took snapshots and listened to the blood vessels, we chatted about the weather getting warmer and how fun NYC can be in the summer. I think she was more excited than I was to have someone closer to her age to talk to.

I waited another 10-15 minutes for Dr. Qao. He came in young, confident, and bold. He sat down and shared that everything sounded and looked pretty good. "Blood flow is normal in the vein now... We couldn't get a good image of the spot where the clot was, but the flow tells us you're okay. We want to keep you on the daily Eliquis for another six months or so though, just as a precaution. Come back and see me in six months and then we can talk about taking you off Eliquis if things continue in this direction." I asked him a few questions before he left, then I walked to checkout to schedule my next appointment: November 21st. *I really hope this is all behind me by then*, I thought. I left the hospital and made my way down to Midtown.

It had been a month since I'd seen Dr. Ari. In his methodical voice and movements, he checked the JP drain and the resection with a rectal exam. I winced and gritted my teeth as usual, but all the pain I had suffered over the last year had made me tougher than I had ever been in my life. I'd figured out how to guard my mind against the pain. *It's all temporary,* I told myself. *It doesn't last long, and then it's gone.*

He asked about the Foley and I gave him a quick "it's still there" answer because I didn't want to talk about it. There was nothing I could do about it, so why was everyone continuing to ask? I had been doing really well, then Dr. Gill had checked the drain and pushed the fluid around; I'd felt like I had the day I'd woken up in recovery post-surgery. I was mad at him but I knew it was irrational. He had done the best he could do, but he was technically the reason I had both of those bags on my legs. I needed someone to blame although there was really no one. Dr. Ari had saved my life but had also put my life in the balance. That was a relationship that was hard to quantify feelings for, *but everything happens for a reason*, I told myself.

I asked Dr. Ari, "When can the drain be removed?"

"We need to proceed with caution and give the hole time to heal and completely close up. I want to see you back in about three weeks." I let the translation sink in. That meant I needed to have the tube in for almost another month—to sleep and sit on one side of my body for three more weeks, to smell the scent of abscess fluid for another three weeks. That was my new normal.

A few weeks went by and I moved from hopeful to depressed, depending on the day. I was walking outside more because I couldn't sit in the apartment any longer, though it didn't take away the fact that every day I had to stare at tubes hanging from my body and I could get winded from just standing too long. Or that I had accidents because my digestive track and bowels weren't fully awake yet. Or the fact that I had sudden stabbing pains in my abdomen and was trying to guess what they could be.

I finally worked up the courage to call my boss and coworkers. As I talked, I either got an "OMG, I don't know what to say; that's terrible" or a "Jesus Christ, Crystal. I'm so sorry." I tried to be optimistic on the phone even though I knew there was no way I could sit at my desk and work the way I used to any time soon. After nearly two months, I could only sit up for about an hour before I was exhausted. But the pain of pity hurt more than anything else. It made me want to get stronger and tougher. *Embrace the pain*, I told myself. *This too shall pass.* I needed to pull myself together.

One weekend, Allen went to visit his mom and I stayed home. I don't even know what we argued about but I knew it was because of my depression. I walked around Brooklyn that day for hours. I lost my balance a few times, but didn't fall. I kept walking until I ran into a festival about 10 blocks away from the apartment. There were people everywhere selling their home country flags. There was music, children dancing, and the scent of grills and food being made with love. I watched until I got too tired to keep standing. I walked across the street to find a place to sit and listened to the music for a while, soaking up the sun. After I'd rested enough, I grabbed my bags from inside my pockets and made my way back home. I apologized to Allen the next day. I knew I was taking my frustrations out on him and that wasn't fair at all. I just wanted to be well again. I was doing all the right things. The old folks used to say, "Do right and right will follow." I'm not so sure I believe that as strongly as I once did.

The next week, I got a UTI. I'd had one or two UTIs in the first 30 years of my life and that was my second UTI in a month. I called the urologist and the receptionist said, "I'm sorry, but Dr. Roberts is on vacation for the next week."

"It's urgent. I am pretty sure I have another UTI."

"Okay, I'll give him the message and he will give you a call."

The urologist called me within an hour and told me he would call in another prescription of Macrobid to my pharmacy. "Take it and if you're not better in a week, give me a call."

I took the medicine and wondered, *how does he know it's going to work?* Maybe urologists always prescribe the same drugs. Each day became more of a struggle towing the line between sorrow and breakthrough.

The next day, I decided I needed to let out some steam and fight the funk I was in. I went to the closet and pulled out my running shoes. I got dressed and headed downstairs to the gym. It had been months since I'd been in there and some faces and machines were new, but the treadmills were still where I last saw them. I gently stepped onto the treadmill and grabbed both sides to lean forward and stretch my legs. I needed to get faster. I didn't recognize myself at all. I was too slow.

I put in my earbuds and turned on the treadmill. I made it to 1 MPH. Anything past 1 MPH and my legs didn't keep up, so I stuck with it. For the next few days, I walked down to the gym and increased the speed on the treadmill just one click at a time. I was feeling motivated and knew I would live again. Until Tuesday.

The following Tuesday, I woke with pain in my abdomen—a different kind of pain. I walked to the bathroom and went through the usual routine; however, this time, when I poured the urine out of my Foley bag, it looked cloudy. *Think Crystal. What does this mean?* It hit me. I had an infection. My temperature felt elevated, my stomach hurt, and my pee was cloudy. I chuckled to myself and beat my fist against the sink. I couldn't catch a break right now! I screamed in the mirror. I didn't cry because I didn't have many tears left. I made my way back to the room to find my phone and called Dr. Le. She said I needed to call Dr. Roberts and probably drop off a urine sample. "The catheters can increase the risks of infection, but you'll be okay," she said.

I called Dr. Roberts and he called me back later in the morning and told me he'd called in a script for Macrobid. "No big deal. Take the Macrobid, and if it doesn't clear up, just call me."

I waited outside for the pharmacy notification message. I walked into Target, picked up the meds, and headed back home. I opened the meds and popped the pill. Little did I know that would be the first of a series of infections to come.

The UTI cleared up and I was continuing to improve each day. I was getting faster on the treadmill and starting to add some weights to my routine. I won't be running another marathon anytime soon, but I was closer to walking at a normal pace again.

After a few days, it was time for my appointment with Dr. Le. I woke that morning, took some pain meds for breakfast, finished my routine, and walked out of the door completely covered in all-black, frumpy, thick clothing because I was freezing though it was 70 degrees out.

I eased into an Uber and headed uptown. I checked in and tried to sit as comfortably as I could, but my body was still rebounding from the IR visit and the recent infection. Dr. Le came in and patted my shoulder. "Crystal, I'm so sorry. Things will get better. They have to, right? ...Here, let me pull up the video so you can see just how deep we had to go to get to the nodule." I didn't really know what I was looking at, but I appreciated her efforts to explain the gravity of my situation and how bad the endo was.

"Now, let's take a look at the Foley. You know, we can teach you how to self-cath. It's not ideal at all, I know, but we can teach you right here in the office today if you want to get rid of the Foley. That would be one less attachment you'd carry around." *Self-cath? As in, do it myself?* The thought of Welan came flooding back to me. I let out a long sigh and tried not to cry.

I had to be strong but the thought of it was terrifying. "I'll consider it if you think it's the right thing to do. I am going to see Dr. Roberts after this, I'll let you know what he says."

"I'd recommend trying, just to improve your quality of life a bit... Let me check your incisions... Great, they are healing up nicely. When do you see Dr. Ari again?"

"Next week."

"Okay, good. Your bladder will come back, these things take time. I'm sorry. I know it's not fun, but you will get through it. You've been through a lot. Call me if you need anything."

"Thank you for everything," I managed to utter. I held my ribcage and inched out of the office. I took a deep breath and walked to the corner. I needed to see Roberts next. I made my way down Fifth Avenue between the buildings and Central Park. It took me a while, but I finally arrived and immediately sat down.

"Do you want to start self-cathing?" asked Dr. Roberts. "I think it's time to remove this so you can go on with your life. We can show you how to do it in the office."

"Um... Okay," I said, reluctantly. My shoulders tightened. I needed to give it a shot. I trusted Dr. Le. If she thought I could do it, I could.

The assistant returned with a blue bag with a logo on the front. Inside were catheters, a mirror, and other supplies for the process.

"Okay," said Dr. Roberts, "let's take the catheter out and then we'll teach you how to do it."

They proceeded to remove the catheter and tossed everything in a small trashcan.

"Okay, I want you to stand up." The assistant grabbed my arm to help me up. I stood on the step of the exam table. "Now pop on the gloves here... Okay, now take your dominant hand and hold the catheter. This is how you'll prepare everything... You can reuse these if you need to, until your supply comes in. You're going to call the number in the bag to place an order. Just sterilize them and let them dry... Now, take your dominant hand and hold the catheter and use the mirror to guide you to the urethra opening."

I fumbled a few times, sweating from the stress, the pain of trying, and standing. After a few attempts and deep breaths, I found my urethra. Urine rushed into the cup the assistant held below the catheter.

"Great. Now you've got the hang of it," said Dr. Roberts.

I felt relief and terror all at once. "The bag is yours to keep," said Dr. Roberts. "Just remember to call the number on the card and place an order," he said, exiting the room.

"Okay, thank you so much for everything," I said to the assistant.

"Ah, same to you, as well," she replied, exiting the room and closing the door behind her.

I gathered my things and looked around the room. My eyes landed on the trashcan. I stared at the catheter bag and tubing. That was the end of that chapter and the start of a new one. I took a deep breath, opened the door, and walked out of the office and into the sunshine. I felt lighter, but the pit of my stomach hurt. I dreaded the next time my bladder would feel full. I tried to stay calm and changed the subject in my mind. *What should I eat for dinner?*

Dread. *What book should I read when I get home?* Terror. Finally in the taxi, I opened the bag and picked up every item to get familiar with it. Allen was in London and my mom was flying in to stay with me for the week. There was a handful of catheters, wipes, gloves, a mirror, and a business card. I called the number to place my first order.

Later that day, my mom arrived. We had dinner and caught up. I told her about the self-cathing and she said, "It's only temporary, Crystal. We just have to do what we have to do to make it." She gave me a soft kiss and patted my arm. To calm my jitters, I told her about a show I'd been watching and I put it on Netflix so she can watch it too. She got into the show. I told her I was tired and was going to get ready for bed. I hadn't had anything to drink and my palms were sweating the entire time. I wiped them on my pants and paced a bit in my room. I needed to have a setup.

I walked into my closet and closed the door. I cleared the floor and placed a towel below the supply bag. I gently laid each supply out so I could prepare myself mentally for each step. I placed the pieces neatly on a towel, then sat on the hard floor and stared at them. I could feel my bladder getting full, and with only a drop coming out, I needed to self-cath soon.

I lay in bed and tried to forget about it. I lay on one side and began to sweat profusely. I got up, paced, and tried to slow my breathing. I had to try.

The room was dark now, with only the city lights in the backdrop and the light on in my closet. I walked into the closet and walked out. In and out. I finally walked in and blew all the air out of my lungs. "I can do this," I whispered. I sanitized my hands and guided the right glove on first. I looked at the sweat beads on my left hand, wiped it, and placed the glove over it. Another deep breath. I opened the catheter package and grabbed the gel. I lifted the catheter, placed the gel in the plastic, and coated the catheter. I was completely naked. Me and my JP drain. With the mirror on the floor, and after forcing my hands steady, I looked for the urethra through the mirror, but my hand was blocking the view. I tried to move the mirror. I couldn't see a thing. I swore under my breath. I poked myself a few times and bottled up the pain. I didn't know how I was going to do this. I lay down and tried to look for it that way, but I couldn't see without putting pressure on the JP drain. I tried and failed again and again. After nearly an hour, I figured out the right arrangement for lighting, the mirror, my body, and the canister position. I prayed. *God, please help me.* I tried two more times. On the third attempt, I did it. I grabbed the canister and placed it below the catheter and the urine began to come out. The sound of the urine hitting the canister was such a relief, my body instantly began to collapse. I held on to the wall and take deep breaths. Once I thought all urine was out, I removed the catheter and placed it back in the plastic it came from. I looked at it and saw blood. *What did I do? Did I damage myself?* I placed a cover over the canister and lay on the floor next to my supply kit and cried. I now had to do this to stay alive. I couldn't let urine back into my kidneys because they would fail. *It could be worse, Crystal. You will live.* I put on a t-shirt and crawled into bed. *If I did it before, I can do it again.* I meditated on those thoughts until I fell asleep. Before dawn, I woke up and I did it again. This time it didn't take an hour; it took about thirty minutes. I came out of the room and dumped the canisters in the toilet. Having my mom there was a much-needed distraction. She was watching the news and resting on the sleeper sofa. I sat on the edge of the bed and asked, "What do you want to do for breakfast?"

While eating breakfast, my mom received a phone call. A family member battling Alzheimer's had passed away. The service would be Saturday. My mom was supposed to stay for the week, but she packed up.

"I wish I could go too," I told her.

"Not yet, my love," she replied, "Soon enough."

The day she left, I decided to go into the city and roam around. I went to Macy's on 34th Street and explored.

A few days passed and Allen was back from London. I wanted to hear all about his trip and how it had went. Those days, it felt like everyone was moving except for me. I felt stuck. Trapped. I still had a drain in my bottom causing one side of my body to get weaker and the other side to get stronger. Then I snapped out of it and told myself I was getting stronger and stronger. I chose life.

I felt something wasn't quite right with the way my urologist was handling my care, so I decided to find a new doctor. He gave me prescriptions but didn't ask for urine samples. He gave me a handful of samples that, based on what I was reading, shouldn't last over a day. I didn't know much about the process, but that didn't feel right. I found another practice in the heart of Midtown and quickly scheduled an appointment for the first available opening.

A week after my final visit to Dr. Roberts and starting my self-cathing journey, I meet with Dr. Johnson in his office, which overlooked parts of Midtown from the sixth floor. He was warm and kind as I told him my story.

He gave me the *wow you've been through quite a bit* speech. He asked lots of questions that I answered as best I could—about the surgery, the previous urologist, and he asked if I had culture results. "You need a healthy supply of catheters. I have a box of samples I can give you. They are very discreet and easier to use, from what I hear. Do not reuse catheters. If you feel you are having an infection, come by the office and drop off a urine sample and we'll culture it to make sure we are giving you the appropriate antibiotics. Sound good?" He patted my shoulder and sent me on my way. I was so happy I had found him.

On the Fourth of July, Allen and I decided to try out a new food hall that had opened last month in DUMBO. We made our way down and walked around the food hall. I was happy to be outside. I checked out all of the restaurants and settled for a good plain burger. Plain with lots of fries! I'd lost weight in places I didn't know one could lose weight. If I ate at all, it was mainly vegan because of the irrational fear that the endo would come back and take me out for good next time.

We returned home so I could rest and have a drink on the rooftop while watching the sun go down. The weather was perfect, and we could see the fireworks show from the rooftop. We watched as fireworks went off on Staten Island, throughout neighborhoods in Brooklyn and Queens, and we could see parts of Manhattan. What a lovely day.

The next week, I get my first visitor. My friend Lilia came over to visit me and brought a lovely bouquet of roses. We sat and talked for about an hour about women's health and how women were walking around every day with a story to tell about their health and healthcare experiences. I asked her many questions about work and her pregnancy. It was a welcome reprieve from my usual routine. We gave each other the biggest hug and parted ways at the elevator. I'll be forever grateful for that small gesture of kindness.

A week later, we received more sad news. Allen's dad passed away on Friday, July 19th. That event snapped me out of thinking about myself and, instead, thinking about Allen and what he needed right now as my partner. The entire time, he had been juggling seeing me in the hospital or hearing insane stories about my recovery, while simultaneously visiting his dad and talking to specialists, doctors, and hospice teams. After his father's stroke in the middle of the courthouse, he had been deemed to be in a vegetative state and wouldn't recover. Allen and I felt his father could hear everything going on around him and when he heard he wasn't going to get better and that he'd be transported to a new home for long-term care, he'd said *no way, man, I'm out of here* and given up his fight. I lost my father when I was 18 years old. I know what it's like to see your flesh and blood in that state. My father, although we weren't close, had an aneurysm episode and was also in a vegetative state until I decided he shouldn't live that way and asked for him to be taken off life support. It's the kind of thing that sticks with you.

Allen's sister set the arrangements for the service. We drove to the Bronx to go through his things and retrieve items Allen wanted to keep. One of Allen's best friends drove up to support him during such a difficult time. I'm forever grateful for that.

After the service, I could see a weight lifted from Allen. He was lighter but heavier. You don't lose a parent and not feel that way. Our lives forever changed in a millisecond. I couldn't help but think about what was next for me. His dad had gone into the hospital the same day I had. *What will my ending look like?* Only time will reveal it.

The next week was the first time in a while that I began to feel like myself again. My hair was growing. My body was getting stronger, and my energy was improving. It had been over two months since the JP drain procedure. I was starting to sleep on my back again with a pillow under my left butt cheek for extra cushion. It was definitely not the most comfortable position, having my spine twisted for 65 days to accommodate, but I could feel we were coming to the end. The tube was now mirky and there wasn't much fluid to be emptied from the bulb anymore. My belly felt close to normal again.

I needed to see Dr. Ari at the end of that week. It had been a little over a month since my last visit. I went to his office with a little more confidence this time. His demeaner was different when he saw me. I must have looked terrible before because, now, he was smiling. I told him that almost all of my symptoms had subsided. There wasn't much coming out of the tube anymore, so I wasn't sure if it was blocked again or if the abscess was gone. Dr. Ari checked the tube and, this time, he didn't do a rectal exam. *Hallelujah!* "Based on your symptoms subsiding and how you look and feel, we can take the drain out today if you like," he said.

My head jerked forward and my eyes grew wide. "You mean in here? Today? I don't have to go back to the hospital for that?"

"No, no, I can take it out here in the office."

"Oh, well, um ... whew. What are the risks?"

"Well, the risk is that the leak hasn't fully healed yet, there is a chance of that, although I think it's probably okay by now."

I paused for a minute. *Wow, I could be free of this tube right here, right now? I don't know. I don't want to have to go back to the hospital for the drain to be reinserted. What should I do?* The familiar was less scary. "Let's keep in it for now." I hated those words coming out of my mouth, but I didn't want to get sick again.

"Ok, no problem. Come back and see me in a few weeks and we can have this conversation again." Dr. Ari waved his hand and nodded his head as he grabbed sanitizer and left the room. Even though the tube was not gone, a weight had been lifted: I didn't have to go back to the hospital to have it removed. I practically skipped out of the office and called my mom to tell her the good news; I sent Allen a text. They were both excited for me. It was about time.

The next day, Allen and I decided to meet in the city for pizza. We met in Downtown Manhattan at one of our favorite pizza places. We only went there once or twice a year because I had cut almost all dairy out of my diet after my diagnoses. I was so excited and ready to live a normal life again; I was so close. We took the train downtown and walked over to our pizza spot. After our first date, five years ago, we had taken Citi bikes from midtown to downtown and stopped there for lunch. I remembered that being my first true NYC pizza experience. Now, I had a fresh start and nothing could get in the way of my happiness. I savored every single sip and bite.

13

THE SUN WILL SHINE AGAIN

August 1, 2019. I woke up and took the Q train to the last Brooklyn bound stop, to Coney Island in the middle of the day when it was slow and I didn't have to worry about my pace. I looked around for a while and walked right back to the Q train, hopped on, and headed back to Downtown Brooklyn.

I try to do things that bring me peace and joy every single day now. I practice being mindful of the blessing that is life because, at any moment, it could end. I refused to waste it.

Day 80 since ER Visit

I took the train to Midtown and visited Dr. Ari to determine if the JP drain should be removed. As usual, I signed in and sat in the lobby. The ladies knew me on a first-name basis by then. They told me it would be just a minute, one of them would come for me soon. I felt excited but nervous. They called me back and told me Dr. Ari would be in shortly. After a minute, he came in and we exchanged pleasantries. "Is today the day?" I asked him.

"Well, let's check it out and see... There isn't much coming out of the tube at all anymore. We can take it out today or you can wait another two weeks and come back."

"I don't know." I was nervous because I couldn't afford another ER visit to Lenox Hill. I told him, "Let's just keep it in."

"Okay, whatever makes you most comfortable."

I left the room and, as I was checking out, I abruptly told the nurse, "I've changed my mind, I want to take it out today. It's time."

I was scared and excited all at once. The drain had saved my life but it was time for us to part ways. I was terrified at my own words, but felt it was the right thing to do. I could no longer wallow in fear. It was time to start living again. The doctor came back in and asked, "Are you sure?"

I decisively told him, "Yes. Final answer."

"Okay," he said with a grin and nod. "I'll be right back."

The nurse came in and helped me lower my undies. I lay on my stomach and took a deep breath. The doctor returned, slapped on some gloves, and laid out some medical gear. "You will likely feel some pressure and pain, but nothing you can't handle," he said. I clutched the medical table and squeezed tightly. He started to remove the medical grade tape around the tube, then he lifted the tube and sterilized the area. He tugged and tugged for what was only a few seconds but felt like forever. I winced and held on and, just like that, the tube was gone. My exhale was one of relief and excitement. Milestones usually consist of graduations, weddings, and childbirth—not this one. Not mine. This was monumental. After 80 agonizing days, the tube was gone.

They cleaned and dressed the area with some gauze and a band aid, and helped me sit up. "That's it?" I asked.

"That's it. It's out. You may see a small amount of discharge from the incision as it's healing. You know to call us if you feel anything like you did before."

I politely thanked him for everything. He smiled and left. I touched my side and my left cheek. Nothing was there. I could sit on both butt cheeks for the first time in 80 days. That chapter was closed.

I checked out for the last time, thanked the staff, and walked out the door. I didn't look back. I smiled all the way out of the building and stepped out into the summertime breeze. I stood for a moment with the sun on my face and recalled the first time I'd come to the building for a consult. One hundred days later, here I was. It was finally over. I could feel it in my soul. This was, oddly, shaping up to be one of the best days of my life.

The symbolism of what that day stands for, I'll never forget.

I took one last look at the building and slid my earbuds in. With extra vigor, I walked back to the subway station and hopped on the train. I stood this time, the way I used to do, and my heart felt like it might burst with excitement. I had a new thrill for life and living it. I sent my family a text to share the good news. When I got home, I put my favorite song on repeat and danced. I danced until I was out of breath, and when I caught my breath, I danced some more. As long as my legs and body allowed movement, I danced. My cheeks hurt from smiling and laughing. *I made it*, I thought. I cried again, but this time, the tears were Hope Tears. Somehow, someway, I was alive!

14

DOVES
AND RAINBOWS

It's been four years, almost to the day, since my 2nd laparoscopic surgery. I wrote this book during my journey and I debated whether to write an epilogue, but felt it was imperative for you, the reader, to know what happened next, if there is a happy ending.

Shortly after Day 80, Allen and I packed up the car and he drove us down to Atlanta for a fresh start. It took me another month or so to feel as though I'd recovered from the surgery. I had to rebuild the side of my body I hadn't used for over 80 days because of the JP drain. I had to eat a clean diet and slowly add in more exercise.

After getting settled, Allen and I agreed we needed to explore our options for starting a family. I began meeting with local reproductive endocrinologists and settled on the perfect place for us. After a few ultrasounds and tests, I sat in the RE's office one day and she told me that, based on my history, it was highly unlikely I would ever get pregnant naturally and my odds were 1 in 4, at best, in ever getting pregnant via IVF. I was unphased by the news. I'd heard it all and this certainly couldn't break me after all I'd been through. I remember thinking to myself: *I will have a baby. I will. I survived endo. Faith over fear.*

The doctor's job was to be truthful and honest about my odds, but in the end, Allen and I defied them. We went through one round of IVF and I was pregnant. I was fortunate because I skipped the part where you need to provide proof to insurance providers that you need IVF. I had enough proof and then some. As a result, we were able to go through our IVF journey right before COVID-19 shut down the world. There are so many families who weren't so lucky.

On October 27, 2020, after many drugs, needles, tests, and a healthy pregnancy, my daughter was born. I had a C-section because, after everything I had gone through, no doctor in their right mind would allow me to attempt a natural labor and delivery. I heard my daughter cry for the first time in the operating room and I cried more tears, but they were tears of joy this time. After my doctor finished sewing me up, she peeked through the curtain and said, "Crystal, I looked at your fallopian tubes like you asked and they are mangled."

Two years later, after running around all weekend with my one-year-old daughter, I crashed on the bed, closed my eyes, and thought to myself, *I don't feel well. Something feels different.* I went to the bathroom and pulled out an old pregnancy test from nearly two years ago. *There is no way I'm pregnant because I don't have functioning fallopian tubes. The HSG proved it and my*

GYN saw it with her own eyes. My tubes were mangled, she said! The test was positive. I took another test. I was pregnant. I laughed hysterically and stared at the tests for a while. God made us laugh that day. I didn't truly believe it until the first ultrasound.

On October 11, 2022, my son was born. Both of my babies are the definition of miracles.

Now, I'm a mom of two and I cherish every second I have with them on this earth. The joy I have seeing them happy and healthy is something words cannot describe. I'd love to say that that was the end and I lived happily ever after, but that wouldn't be accurate. The first year after my traumatic incidents were tough. I struggled to keep my composure when talking about what had happened. I had several doctors tell me I should see a therapist to talk about my grief and trauma. After surviving endo, life is a constant game of staying positive and looking at the bright side.

When I moved to Atlanta, I immediately found a new urologist (#3). He recommended that I take a drug to help prevent UTIs and if I think I have a UTI, to drop off a urine sample. His office was a bit too busy, and it became increasingly difficult to speak to or see anyone, so, within a few months, I found another doctor—urologist #4.

Number 4 seemed to be the perfect fit. He was the first to give me a proper game plan. He was the first to introduce me to UDS (urodynamics study). He got me through both pregnancies. During both pregnancies, I suffered from chronic UTIs due to the catheters. I couldn't take just any antibiotics and I certainly couldn't take any medicines to prevent them. I had to be sent to an infectious disease doctor during the last trimester of both pregnancies for alternative treatment.

After my daughter was born, he had talked to me about trying out the bladder pacemaker, a device that sends signals to the brain that tells your body to urinate. After a list of questions, I agreed. There would be two surgeries required. The first would be to install the test device (to see if it was worth moving forward with the permanent implant). The test was installed. I felt I was seeing results, so I went ahead with the permanent, but it didn't quite work out like I'd hoped.

During my 2nd pregnancy, I got the pacemaker removed because it started to move and poke out a bit. I could feel the implant moving around and it left me with debilitating pain whenever I tried to walk. I had the device and sacral nerve stimulation (SNS) lead removed via outpatient surgery with only topical anesthesia due to pregnancy risks. This was my first and last time being awake in an operating room with no anesthetics! I could hear everything the team was saying and felt the implant being ripped out of my body. I could feel the knife cutting back the skin layers to get the battery pack out of my butt cheek. Sadly, endometriosis prepared me for this type of pain. There were three more surgeries (outpatient) in less than two years after my endo excision and rectal resection. More scars left behind...

When my son was about four months old, I realized I had a UTI and slowly made my way over to drop off a urine sample. Something happened to the sample and they called and asked me to bring another the very next day. I did. I felt no symptoms, but there was cloudy urine. I began to feel achy and sick by the weekend and knew it was the UTI. The next morning, I went to urgent care for treatment, but it was too late. My body started to react in ways I'd never seen it react before. I broke out in hives and my body began to swell. I drove myself to the ER the next morning and they swore I had a food allergy. I was told to drink water to flush it out. I asked them to draw blood to test for sepsis because I had seen this movie before. They brushed me off and told me it couldn't be that. Thank God, it wasn't. It took a few weeks to recover after the mountain of meds they had prescribed, including a steroid for swelling that had nothing to do with a true allergic reaction.

I saw an allergist two weeks later. He said it was my body's way of responding under stress and that I did not develop a food allergy. By then, I already knew this as well, but needed to get it confirmed. I had to stop breast-feeding by force so I could get back on a medication regimen. Being forced to stop when I was not ready to crushed me—and weening comes with its own set of issues and hormonal changes. That was my second ER visit due to a severe UTI.

I went to see my urologist a few days later. What he said cut deep, but I hid the pain of his words. He said, "What am I going to do with you? As a specialist, my job is to fix something so I can release you back to the care of the one who sent you." I knew then that he'd given up on me. I knew I needed to find #5. Instead, I decided to go and see a Pelvic Floor Physical Therapist. It was one of the best health decisions I'd made in a while.

During our second session, the physical therapist said, "I really think you should get a second opinion. I know a urogynecologist that is wonderful and believes in a team approach to healthcare."

I went to see her the very next week. Number 5 examined me and listened to my story. She suggested that we perform a pelvic exam, another UDS (urodynamics study), a renal scan, and a cystoscopy. I was in her office once a week for a month, a different test each time.

This is the slimmed down version of the aftermath, but I share it so you can get an idea of how much time, energy, and financial resources endo has cost me.

After all this, the good news is that I survived endometriosis. I am completely pain free now. I know that with faith, support, and time, I will make a *full* recovery.

Writing this, it sounds like what happened to me is horrible, but you see, I've become the woman I was always supposed to be. I had many fears while writing this book. Fear of embarrassment. Fear of criticism. Fear that strangers and my family and friends would never look at me the same once they knew the whole story. But the fear of not sharing my story, even if it only touched one person, kept me up at night. That fear motivated me far beyond the fear of what people may think of me.

Deep Infiltrating Endometriosis (DIE) wanted me to die, but I refused. Despite it all, I am determined to fly high and enjoy the life God has given me.

Endometriosis tried to leave me with deep physical, mental, and emotional wounds and scars, but none of that matters anymore. I did not quit. I choose to count each blessing and seek the little things to be grateful for in this life.

I felt led by God to write and share this book on April 3, 2019. I thought I had a story to share, but that was only the beginning. There are so many women who have stories far more painful than mine. By amplifying our voices, we can prompt changes in medical schools, legislation, and pharmaceuticals, and help lessen the impacts to the young women coming behind us. I had to go through the pain to be inspired to write my story. I hope you tell yours or advocate on behalf of those who cannot tell theirs. I hope and pray that, in twenty years, endometriosis is no longer an issue because we will have the knowledge to prevent the disease, and better natural and medical solutions to heal our bodies. Until that day, hang on to hope and know you are not alone. Let's *live*.

ABOUT THE AUTHOR

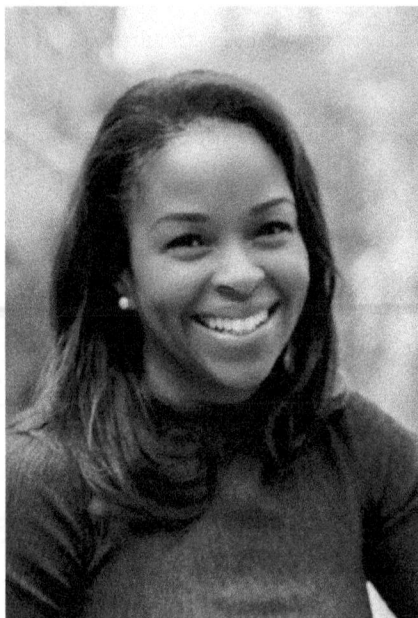

C rystal Brown was born in Birmingham, Alabama. She studied psy-
chology and business administration at the University of Alabama
and has a master's degree in business administration from Emory
University. Crystal never dreamed of writing a memoir but began recording
her healing journey six months after her diagnosis.

Crystal enjoys spending time with family, reading, watching movies,
baking (thanks to her mom), and running.

www.ingramcontent.com/pod-product-compliance
Lightning Source LLC
Chambersburg PA
CBHW030016290326
41934CB00005B/358